ONCOLOGY CRITICAL CARE

Edited by **Jeffrey B. Hoag**

Oncology Critical Care
http://dx.doi.org/10.5772/61590
Edited by Jeffrey B. Hoag

Contributors
Emil Abramian, Trisha Patel, Mashiul Chowdhury, Erica McGovern, Denise Wolfe, Mark Lewis, Jeroen Van Vugt, Audrey Jongen, Victor Van Woerden, Elisabeth De Wijkerslooth De Weerdesteijn, Patrick De Hoogt, Jan Stoot, Juul Tegels, Deepjot Singh, Robert Bonomo, Danish Ahmad, Kellie Joseph, Christopher Halpin

Published by InTech
Janeza Trdine 9, 51000 Rijeka, Croatia

Publishing Process Manager Romina Rovan
Technical Editor SPi Global
Cover InTech Design team

First published December, 2016
Printed in Croatia

Additional hard copies can be obtained from orders@intechopen.com

Oncology Critical Care, Edited by Jeffrey B. Hoag
p. cm.
Print ISBN 978-953-51-2781-9
Online ISBN 978-953-51-2782-6

For EU product safety concerns:
IN TECH d.o.o., Prolaz Marije Krucifikse Kozulić 3, 51000 Rijeka, Croatia, info@intechopen.com or visit our website at intechopen.com.

Meet the editor

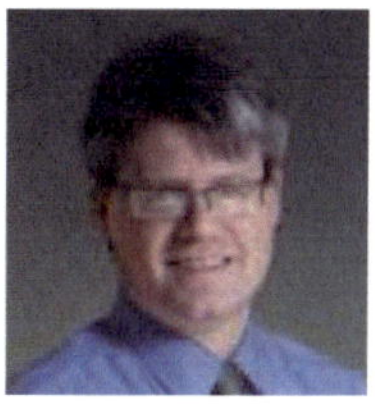

Dr. Jeffrey B. Hoag received his Doctor of Medicine degree from Virginia Commonwealth University School of Medicine in Richmond, Virginia, in 2001. After completing internship and residency in the same institution, he moved to Baltimore, Maryland, where he completed fellowship training at Johns Hopkins University in Pulmonary Medicine and Critical Care Medicine. Along with being an associate professor of Medicine at Drexel University College of Medicine, he is the director of Critical Care at the Eastern Regional Medical Center of Cancer Treatment Centers of America® in Philadelphia, Pennsylvania. Dr. Hoag is also the enterprise chief of Critical Care and vice chairman of Medicine for Medicine and Science, the clinical branch of Cancer Treatment Centers of America®.

Contents

Preface

According to the American Cancer Society, more than 1.6 million people will be diagnosed with cancer during this year (2016), and there will be approximately half a million cancer-related deaths this year in the United States. Outcomes have steadily risen over the last several decades for most cancer types with the advent of newer chemotherapy regimens, improved interventional and surgical techniques, targeted radiation therapies and immunotherapies, as well as earlier diagnostic and screening programs. As outcomes have improved, there are more and more patients with cancer that are developing serious illness. Some of these patients develop critical illness that is not a direct result of their comorbid malignancy; however, a significant number of patients have critical illness that can be directly attributed to their cancer or its treatment.

In the not-too-distant past, patients with active malignancy were thought not appropriate for critical care services as decreased longevity related to the cancer suggested poor prognosis for intensive care utilization. However, more recently, there is evidence supporting rapid activation of critical care services can lead to improved outcomes in patients with cancer. As this subset of critically ill patients presents in greater frequency to critical care physicians, specific knowledge regarding this special group of patients is paramount to appropriate treatment. Moreover, just as sub-subspecialty critical care experience in trauma, neurosciences, and transplant among others has proved beneficial, the emerging field of oncology critical care warrants specific attention.

The following chapters highlight some specific topics of critical illness experienced by patients with cancer with specific focus on the interaction of how the presence of underlying malignancy affects treatment discussions and decisions. Although not exhaustive, these topics provide details of respiratory, gastrointestinal, infectious, nutritional, and pharmacological issues in critically ill patients with cancer. I truly appreciate the dedication and involvement of this group of authors not only in the development of this work but also in the care they provide to their patients.

Jeffrey B. Hoag, MD, MS
Director of Pulmonary and Critical Care, Eastern Regional Medical Center
Vice Chairman, Department of Medicine, Medicine and Science
Cancer Treatment Centers of America®
Philadelphia, USA

Chapter 1

Oncological Airway Emergencies in the Critical Care Unit

Osheen Abramian, Diana Kolman and
Emil Abramian

Additional information is available at the end of the chapter

http://dx.doi.org/10.5772/65082

Abstract

Malignancies involving the upper and lower airways can be presented as acute and/or acute-on-chronic life-threatening emergencies. Most of them require intensive care unit (ICU) admission and acute intervention. Such emergencies include but are not exhaustive to epistaxis, massive hemoptysis, central airways obstruction, postobstructive pneumonia, tracheoesophageal fistula, and pleural disease. These are frequent consequences of disease, iatrogenicity, and various pleural diseases causing respiratory failure. The incidence, physiology, symptoms, and sequelae of each disease will be outlined in addition to potential surgical, pharmacologic, and conservative interventions. An anatomical approach from the upper airway, lower airway, mediastinum, and pleura will be taken. Here, we discuss interventions such as emergent cautery, nasal packing, emergent airways, and tracheostomy in addition to a brief glance at other surgical modalities. We will also detail central airway complications such as obstructing endobronchial tumors, massive hemoptysis, bronchoscopy, rigid bronchoscopy, stent placement, and other interventions (cautery, cryotherapy, one-way valves). Finally, pleural disorders such as tension pneumothorax, bronchopleural fistulas, massive pleural effusion, and hemothorax will be reviewed.

Keywords: respiratory failure, central airway obstruction (CAO), upper airway obstruction, epistaxis, massive hemoptysis, stridor, endoluminal disease, malignant pleural effusion, massive pleural effusion, tension pneumothorax, hemothorax, bronchopleural fistula, ENT, interventional pulmonology, cardiothoracic surgery, thoracotomy, thoracostomy, intrapleural fibrinolysis

1. Introduction

As the armamentarium of oncologists continues to improve, so do the outcomes of their patients. However, morbidity persists and many patients require intensive care unit (ICU) as a consequence of end-stage disease, multiorgan dysfunction, infection, and airway compromise. This chapter focuses on airway emergencies that are typically experienced in the ICU. Classification and designation of tumors will not be reviewed. Rather yet, the airway and mediastinal burden of tumor will be detailed. We have organized the discussion in an anatomical approach, sequenced as such: upper airway (nasal cavity, pharynx, and larynx), lower airway (trachea, primary bronchi, and parenchyma), and pleura.

1.1. Upper airway obstruction

We consider upper airway obstruction attributable to cancer a medical emergency. The clinical manifestations of airway obstruction will depend on the underlying disease, the anatomic location, acuity, and severity of airway compromise. Primary head and neck tumors causing upper airway obstruction are perilaryngeal tumors including supraglottic, pharyngeal, pyriform fossa, periglottic, vocal cord, and subglottic lesions. Almost all (95%) of head and neck cancers are squamous cell carcinomas [2], and most occur in patients with an extensive smoking history. Obstruction can occur via mass effect, edema, or hemorrhage. Metastatic breast, colon, melanoma, sarcoma, lymphoma, and esophageal cancers are also associated with upper airway obstruction [2]. Certain obstructions can be asymptomatic and can develop insidiously, making propensity to clinical deterioration unpredictable. Airway salvage and maintenance of oxygenation is the main interventional objective. In this chapter, we also emphasize early airway protection and limiting use of paralytics.

1.2. Etiology and pathogenesis

Upper airway obstruction can be classified as functional, anatomic (e.g., squamous cell carcinoma of larynx), acute, or subacute. Based on the site of obstruction, patients can be divided into different subclasses including obstructive lesions in and around the larynx, mid-tracheal obstruction due to retrosternal goiters, and thyroid carcinomas. We highlight a key respiratory physiologic determinant of airway resistance, Poiseuille's Law. Simply put, airway resistance is dependent on airway diameter and turbulence. Thusly, small changes in airway diameter lead to large changes in resistance of the airflow as the airway resistance is directly proportional to the length and inversely proportional to the fourth power of the airway radius [15].

1.3. Diagnosis

If suspected, we suggest an anatomic survey to rule out airway obstruction. Many modalities are available to the intensivist, such as direct laryngoscopy, bronchoscopy, and flouroscopic guidance. Our practice is to evaluate the patient starting cephalad and progressing caudad, both through direct visualization and for establishing a differential diagnosis. Coupling underlying medical history and physical exam with appropriate imaging, the treatment plan should be formulated promptly. With CT imaging of the neck and mediastinal structures, we are able to identify the extension of disease and its positioning relative to nearby anatomy. Routine chest radiography in this sense is limited to its two-dimensional depictions and helps identify tracheal and skeletal abnormalities but mainly helps indicate what next imaging modality is needed.

1.4. Signs and symptoms

We commonly observe symptoms of upper airway obstruction as respiratory distress, hoarseness, stridor, facial swelling, or failure to oxygenate with a bag-valve mask. Supraglottic, subglottic, or cancers of the hypopharynx do not usually cause voice changes and are therefore diagnosed in late stages. The most common cause of hoarseness is edema of the true vocal cords. Six weeks of hoarseness in an adult is highly suspicious for a precancerous or cancerous laryngeal lesion. Although not considered a true emergency, hoarseness warrants thorough evaluation.

Stridor is defined as a high-pitched wheezing heard during the respiratory cycle, and is usually more intense during the inspiratory phase. It is appreciated when the airway is at least 5 mm or 50% of its previous diameter [13, 23]. The most common cancers associated with stridor from airway obstruction are squamous cell carcinoma of the larynx, trachea, and esophagus. Pancoast tumors can secondarily cause interstitial edema of the head and neck leading to airway compromise from superior vena cava (SVC) obstruction.

1.5. Management of upper airway obstruction

The primary objective for an intensivist is to establish and safely provide an airway. Malignancies of the base of the tongue, nasopharynx, pyriform fossa, epiglottis, and vocal cords will usually require a surgical airway such as tracheotomy or cricothyrotomy. These tumors have a high propensity for bleeding and special precautions must be taken and emergent surgical consultation must be considered. If the airway is amenable to intubation, smaller-sized endotracheal tubes should be amenable. Long-acting sedatives and muscle relaxants should be avoided as they predispose airway obstructions to airway collapse and respiratory failure. Long-term definitive management involved treating the underlying cause, which is usually treated surgically. However, the majority of patients with malignant airway obstructions will be unresectable due to locally advanced disease, metastatic disease, or poor surgical candidacy.

2. Epistaxis and Post Operative Hematoma

Epistaxis, or nosebleed, occurs in up to 10% of patients with advanced cancer. Common causes of epistaxis in the cancer population are intranasal neoplasms, polyps, leukemia, and coagulopathic disorders including thrombocytopenia secondary to malignancy, medication, or anticoagulation. It is frequently associated with squamous cell carcinoma, melanoma, and papillomatous lesions [1]. Although rare, nasal cavities can also be a source of metastasis [2].

Epistaxis is anatomically classified as being located in the anterior or posterior nasopharynx. Occasionally, patients might present with severe, life-threatening epistaxis that arises from the larger vessels in the posterior and superior nasal cavity. This bleeding can compromise the airway and results in respiratory failure. Although a thorough medical history and physical exam is necessary, rapid epistaxis can become a life-threatening event. If time allows for quantification of bleeding, the duration and/or a history of a bleeding disorder should be taken into account. Despite the profound incidence of all-cause epistaxis, a societal guideline on management does not exist. Our approach, as in all institutions, is evidence-based nevertheless [3]. A stepwise approach is pertinent and consists of hemostasis conservative measures, localized tamponade, and surgical specialist intervention [4].

2.1. Anterior epistaxis

Patients with active or frequent nosebleeds should be evaluated for an anterior source of bleeding. Approximately 90% of anterior nosebleeds occur at Kiesselbach's plexus or Little's area. As a consequence, most of the blood exits anteriorly. This is supplied from the external carotid artery, the superior labial branch of the facial artery, and the terminal branch of the sphenopalantine artery. The internal carotid also supplies the anterior and posterior ethmoidal arteries.

Visualizing the bleeding with nasal speculum/thudicum with a light source is the initial approach but is inferior to direct rhinoscopy/nasendoscopy [4–6]. If blood obfuscates visualization, irrigation or suctioning techniques should be pursued. Applying direct mechanical pressure may control bleeding, by manually occluding the anterior aspect of the nose in a pincer fashion while leaning forward or applying pressure with an ice pack for 15 min. This serves to tamponade the lesion and allows for platelet aggregation and clot activation. Patients should be kept upright [7].

Nasal packing is a skill that the intensivist should be comfortable in administering while awaiting otolaryngology evaluation. Risk of nasal packing includes but is not limited to tissue necrosis, obstruction, and infection. The anterior nares should be packed with Merocel® tampon or gauze soaked with 4% lidocaine and oxymetazoline to promote vasoconstriction. There is little data, however, showing oxymetazoline's role in hastening hemostasis. Friable lesions causing epistaxis can bleed even more with treatment intervention. If a bleeding vessel is visualized, electrical or chemical cautery (silver nitrate) for hemostasis should be pursued only on lateral nares and not the septum to prevent perforation. Anterior nasal packing should be applied for refractory bleeding. Packing failure can be explained by inadequate placement or anatomic deformity such as a deviated septum or nasal airway obstruction by tumor or polyp. In these patients, a careful endoscopic examination under general anesthesia should be considered. We do not recommend blood pressure reduction for the sole purpose of controlling bleeding. Nevertheless, one must assess signs of hemodynamic instability and necessity of volume resuscitation.

http://dx.doi.org/10.5772/65082

2.2. Posterior epistaxis

Posterior nosebleeds carry the highest risk of significant hemorrhage. Patients with persistent bleeding in spite of conventional treatment should be evaluated for a posterior bleeding source. Approximately 10% of bleeds occur posteriorly, along the nasal septum or lateral nasal wall. The blood supply includes the external carotids through the sphenopalantine branch of the internal maxillary artery. Bleeding enters the nasopharynx and oral cavity, placing the patient at a high risk of respiratory compromise [8, 9]. Concordantly, the management of a posterior bleed is more complicated. Posterior nasal packing is prone to impairing oxygenation. With heavy bleeding, electrocautery and then silver nitrate can aid hemostasis [10]. Both interventions carry a risk of septal perforation; however, electrocautery is easier to apply than silver nitrate during heavy bleeding [11]. It is recommended that an ear, nose, and throat specialist (ENT) be consulted for placement of an inflatable balloon or a 12–14 French Foley catheter for posterior packing.

At times, posterior gauze packs can be introduced through the mouth and retracted back into the nasopharynx, thus providing tamponade in the area of choanae and the sphenopalantine foramen. When conservative measures fail, embolization or surgical ligation of the offending vessel may be necessary. If surgical ligation by an otolaryngologist fails, patients can be referred to an interventional radiologist for angiography and embolization.

2.3. Postoperative neck hematoma

The diagnosis of a postoperative hematoma is based on clinical exam, CT head and neck imaging, and subsequently confirmed with needle aspiration. Hematomas of clinical significance could be presented acutely or in a subacute timeline post procedurally. Obstructions of the airways occur as a consequence of edema and/or direct compression of the airway. An acute presentation requires a focus on airway management, whereas chronic hematomas may be a nidus to infection. If the airway is obstructed, the method of intubation is dictated by the degree of airway edema and extent of previous surgery. Hematomas can also be decompressed by either aspiration or releasing surgical staples. If the hematoma is due to an arterial bleed, it can only be stopped by direct digital pressure or clamping. These patients should be evaluated surgically.

3. Approach to Lower Airway Emergencies

Tumors of the tracheobronchial tree and mediastinum can cause respiratory failure and ICU admission. Although primary tumors of the trachea are rare [12], mediastinal, primary lung, and metastatic lesions can cause a multitude of clinical symptoms. If not addressed promptly, morbidity and mortality can be significant. Diagnostic and therapeutic modalities are now available offering bronchoscopic and, if needed, surgical approaches to expedite and minimize patient complications. Approximately 20–30% of primary lung cancers can be presented with central airway disease and its sequelae [13] such as atelectasis, hemoptysis, central airway obstruction (CAO), and postobstructive pneumonias.

3.1. Hemoptysis

Although some of the most common causes of hemoptysis include bronchitis, bronchiectasis, and airway trauma, we will be focusing on neoplastic causes. The underlying cause is either due to endoluminal disease (primary or metastatic), distal invasive disease (including those of infectious etiology), and coagulopathy or as consequences of systemic disease (i.e., thrombocytopenia and drug induced injury). Approximately 20% of lung cancer patients will experience hemoptysis throughout their disease progression [14] with case series reports of up to 3% having massive hemoptysis [15].

Aside from neoplastic hemoptysis, other causes, such as heart failure, pulmonary tuberculosis, lung abscess, coagulopathic, and iatrogenic (airway interventions) should be in the list of initial differential diagnosis. Hemoptysis is frequently attributable to bronchogenic carcinoma; however, massive hemoptysis is usually due to squamous cell carcinoma (e.g., centrally located tumors) [16].

3.2. Diagnosis and management

Hemoptysis can be presented with clinically insignificant streaks or can be catastrophic. It can include severity that is so burdened by fulminant bleeding that it impairs ventilatory capacity. It is often in these scenarios that require ICU care, if escalation had not already been established.

The initial approach includes quantification of the amount of blood loss as to help assess the risk of respiratory failure and asphyxiation. There is no universally defined volume of hemoptysis to define as massive. However, volumes exceeding 200 cc/h or 600 cc in 24 h [15] are volumes large enough for expeditious diagnostic and therapeutic intervention. In large volume hemoptysis, airway protection becomes paramount and intubation is usually necessary. Regardless of the volume, hemoptysis is clinically considered massive when patients become difficult to ventilate (regardless of underlying morbidity) or if they demonstrate hemodynamic instability [17].

The initial precautions and interventions to massive life-threatening hemoptysis are universal. This includes maintaining head of the bead (HOB)>30 degrees, monitoring for hemodynamic instability, airway protection, and ensuring oxygenation. Patients should be positioned in the dependent position to preserve the nonbleeding lung from pooling or blood spillage. The objective is to identify the source of bleeding. Frequently life-threatening hemoptysis warrants bronchoscopic evaluation with balloon tamponade/endoluminal ablation.

In malignant hemoptysis, chest radiography helps illustrate lunch parenchyma. Aside from identifying masses and cavitations, radiographs are superseded by multidetector CT (MDCT). The CT helps visualize abnormal arteries, information which is critical for possible embolization. While a diagnostic evaluation as to the source includes these investigational modalities, emergent bleeding in the ICU deems a patient too unstable for transport. Should the history and or radiographic imaging not be available, emergent intubation preferably via bronchoscopy should be completed to isolate the nonbleeding bronchus [18]. Nevertheless, identifying the cause of hemoptysis in an emergency should overlap the therapeutic interventions and

http://dx.doi.org/10.5772/65082

must not be a cause of delay. Priority should be taken to identify which lung, or if both, the bleeding is originating from. Admittedly, a medical history and physical exam is not extensively helpful in identifying the location of bleeding. History should thus be succinct and oriented at cardiopulmonary, infectious, coagulopathic, and infectious etiologies.

Attention should be paid to any role in coagulopathy reversal, necessity of blood product transfusion, and assessing oxygenation with blood gas analysis. Moreover, large-volume hemoptysis is a state of volume depletion, and aggressive intravenous fluid replenishment should be considered if clinically feasible. Also, there is no optimal ventilator setting for massive hemoptysis.

3.3. Bronchoscopy

In an emergent setting, patients should be intubated (with a large bore endotracheal tube), especially if patients will inevitably need bronchoscopy. Bronchoscopic evaluation for hemoptysis is often laden with blood and/or clots forming debris that requires the intensivist to retract, clean, and reinsert the bronchoscope. Also, for clearer visualization, large-volume lavage can risk oxygenation, highlighting the importance of keeping a patient intubated. Both flexible and rigid bronchoscopies have a role in massive hemoptysis; however, with a rigid bronchoscope, suctioning capabilities are greater, as are the therapeutic interventions.

Arteriography for persistent hemoptysis is very useful, as embolization of a bleeding artery is often therapeutic [19, 20]. This is completed by an interventional radiologist in a procedure suite. If hemoptysis has temporarily ceased, we remind the reader that CT chest imaging is frequently useful in localizing the source of bleeding. However, patient transfer requires moderate patient stability and can be time consuming. Tagged red blood cell scanning is not useful in the emergent setting. Thoracic surgery consultation should be pursued if bleeding persists despite therapeutic intervention.

Diagnostic bronchoscopy will also aid in identifying any endoluminal/lobar source, thus dictating the necessary intervention. Should a central bleeding lesion be found during the initial survey, isolation of the nonbleeding side (as highlighted earlier) is recommended as to prevent aspiration of blood into normal parenchyma. Insertion of an endoluminal bronchial blocker (Arndt® Blocker) for initial airway tamponade has utility for prevention of such an event [21]. Once the endobronchial blocker is inserted, the balloon should be kept inflated for at least 24 h before assessing rebleeding. In addition to balloon tamponade, other interventions include cold lavage, cryotherapy, and ablative therapy. Topical vasoconstrictors, such as epinephrine, can also be applied to help slow bleeding.

Compared to flexible bronchoscopy, the larger lumen of the rigid bronchoscope facilitates a greater ability to control bleeding while facilitating ablative therapies, and is discussed in a later section in this chapter (see "Central Airway Obstruction: Immediate Bronchoscopic Ablative Therapy"). If an endobronchial blocker is not available, direct bronchoscopic-guided single-lung intubation may be required until further intervention is amenable. This is done by inserting an endotracheal tube in the main stem bronchus of the nonbleeding lung to wall off any blood overflow. Double-lumen intubation allows breaths to be ventilated to both lungs but is tenuous in the rapidly bleeding airway in which insertion and position maintenance are difficult to maintain. Interventional pulmonology consultation is recommended for the aforementioned potential ablative and/or cryotherapy. Transport to the operating room for rigid bronchoscopy is recommended [21]. As a summation, massive hemoptysis is a life-threatening clinical presentation that warrants immediate action and a multidisciplinary approach. Outlook on treatments options would include endoluminal ablation (argon plasma coagulation or Nd:YAG laser), emergent radiation for distal masses, bronchial or pulmonary artery embolization, and/or a combination of all.

4. Approach to Central Airway Obstruction

A central airway obstruction is an airflow obstruction either at the trachea, carina, or main-stem bronchi. For the intensivist, we outline the malignant etiologies, however, there are benign, traumatic, and iatrogenic (e.g., tracheomalacia) causes as well. Admission into the ICU due to CAO is frequently due to an acute-on-chronic decompensation of a compromised airway. Primary lung tumors are the most common causes of central airway obstruction, most commonly with squamous cell carcinoma followed by adenocarcinoma [22]. Malignant causes can also be due to endoluminal, metastatic, lymph node, mediastinal, or, less commonly, nasopharyngeal disease. Further, we will only concentrate on life-threatening acute CAO. Malignant CAO is primarily palliative in the setting of advanced disease.

The CAO occurs through three basic mechanisms. Simply put, the airway is obstructed either by direct invasion, compression, or endoluminal disease. A mixed picture is possible as well. CAO can develop over months to years; however, those that develop acutely can cause catastrophic outcomes. Patient presentation varies on the degree of obstruction. Significant obstruction causing enough luminal narrowing to disrupt airflow is the primary reason for the sensation of dyspnea. Additional signs and symptoms include cough, localized wheezing, respiratory failure, stridor, and postobstructive pneumonia [23]. Consideration must be made about tracheal luminal narrowing at the time of symptoms, such that exertional dyspnea occurs at about 8 mm of narrowing and symptoms at rest occur at 5 mm [22]. Obstruction can occur in primarily three anatomical variations, defined by the location of mass effect.

One should be prompted to consider CAO in difficult to oxygenate patients with an acute onset of wheezing, stridor, or tachypnea. Oxygenation and ventilation should be prioritized and patients must be assessed for the necessity of ventilator support. We recommend pursuit of the establishment of a secure airway before imaging. If airway obstruction is causing almost definite respiratory failure, cricothyrotomy, tracheostomy, or retrograde intubation may be necessary [24, 25]. Often times in the acutely decompensating patient, rigid bronchoscopic intubation although ideal may not be immediately available. Naturally, larger-diameter endotracheal tubes are preferred. Fiberoptic intubation may be of role, although availability is institution dependent [26]. Intervention should thus be focused on airway patency. There is no role of spirometry in the diagnosis of acute CAO. Also, choice of induction anesthesia is an important consideration, as a moderate amount of sedation is usually required for rigid bronchoscopic intubation. When paralytics or heavy sedatives are used, the already compromised airway can further occlude. Preoxygenation in these instances is of prime importance, and at times the addition of a mixture of helium and oxygen (known as heliox) as a bridge to intubation or definitive treatment is useful in providing laminar flow [27]. Overall, we recommend paralytics be used as a last resort as intubation can be irreversibly compromised if the airway is lost.

Decompensation could also occur with acute bleeding, swelling and/or additional secretions occluding an already narrowed lumen. Clinical parameters such as hypoxia and hypercapnia may not be of much guidance and may misdirect clinicians' initial index of suspicion.

Although initial evaluation of a patient's clinical presentation with medical history and physical exam is pertinent, obtaining relevant imaging in addition to bronchoscopic consideration is central to the management of CAO. Chest radiographs are often the first illustrations attained but they provide little information to the depth and complexity of obstruction. Chest CT imaging is the modality of choice for providing detailed anatomical information that plays a relevant role in formulating a management plan.

4.1. Interventional bronchoscopy

The institutional availability of interventional bronchoscopy is expanding, as is the role in acute CAO management. Direct bronchoscopic visualization can preclude CT imaging, as direct visualization may provide an accurate diagnosis and anatomic obstructive characteristics faster. Not only is bronchoscopy diagnostic, it is primarily considered therapeutic for foreign object retrieval and suctioning of secretions or blood [28]. Ost et al. demonstrated that interventional procedures have been shown to have 93% technical success, where 48% of subjects experiencing improved dyspnea, and a 3.9% complication rate (**Table 1**) [29].

Malignant	Nonmalignant
Primary endoluminal carcinoma	Lymphadenopathy
Bronchogenic	Sarcoidosis
Adenoid Cystic	Relapsing polychondritis
Mucoepidermoid	Granulation tissue
Carcinoid	Hamartomas
Metastatic carcinoma	Papillomatosis
Bronchogenic	Airway stents
Renal Cell	Artificial airways
Thyroid	Mucus pluging
Sarcoma	Blood clot
Melanoma	Granulomatos disease
Laryngeal carcinoma	Goiter
Esophageal carcinoma	Webs
Tumors of the mediastinum	
Lymphadenopathy	

Table 1. Diseases causing central airway obstruction.

4.2. Rigid bronchoscopy

A rigid bronchoscope (**Figure 1**) is pivotal for acute intraluminal CAO for stenting, dilation, and coring. There are a plurality of techniques and devices available; however, the objective is universally oriented at airway patency. In addition, interventional procedures for CAO also provide improvement in palliative symptoms such as exercise tolerance and dyspnea [30]. The interventional modalities vary depending on institution, available resources, operator preferences, and location of CAO. Dilation, via balloon or mechanical coring, can be used for both extraluminal and endoluminal tumor burden. Dilation with a rigid bronchoscope can be advantageous as it can also be simultaneously utilized for patient intubation. CAO with high risk of perforation or bleeding may be sequentially dilated.

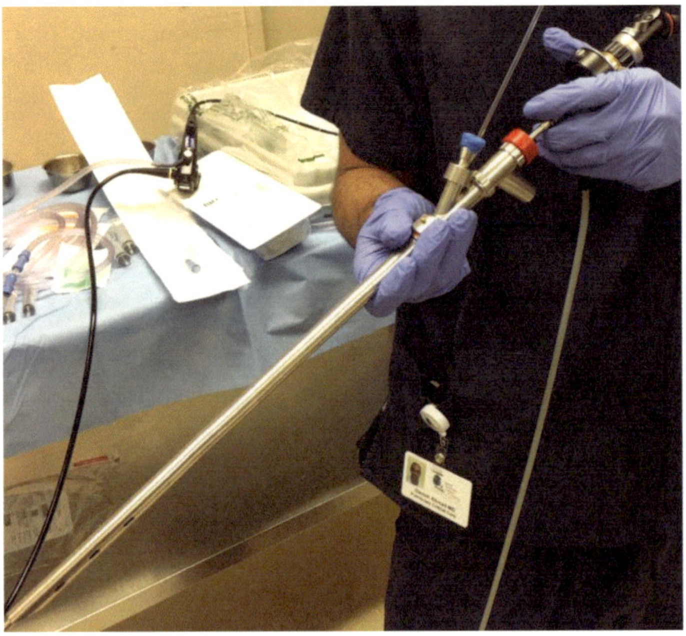

Figure 1. Rigid Bronchoscope (picture courtesy, Emil Abramian MD).

4.3. Immediate bronchoscopic ablative therapy

Immediate ablation is highly effective at clearing CAO. However, ablation usually requires coupling with a second intervention, such as stenting. Ablation primarily consists of argon plasma coagulation (APC) and electrocautery. Extraluminal obstructions are managed with dilation and stenting. These procedures have been found to have similar outcomes, and modality is dependent on the proceduralist's preference [31]. Eventual maintenance of airway patency is usually obtained by multiple interventional approaches (e.g., tumor coring and subsequent stenting) [28]. Reopening of the airway (>50%) was achieved in the majority of cases in a recent multicenter study [29].

Laser therapy (Nd:YAG, argon, excimer) is a promptly effective therapy for intraluminal CAO; however, it is not suitable for long lesions (>4 cm). Laser ablation essentially results in destruction of the obstructing vascularizing vessels and ends with subsequent obstruction extraction. Electrocautery is an alternative to laser therapy but the direct thermal administration causes a risk for airway fire, and is only suitable for endoluminal disease.

Argon plasma coagulation (APC), another noncontact thermal ablative, is highly effective for vascular lesions with a high tendency to bleed, or those that are nestled in airway bifurcations. In contrast to laser therapy, argon gas is electrically coupled to create electrical current that creates target tissue destruction through a grounding principle. As such, flat lesions and lesions at airway bifurcations that are difficult to visualize are effectively managed with APC. The naturally coagulant effects of argon are also advantageous for achieving hemostatis. Moreover, obliteration of granulation tissue surrounding metallic stents is safely approached with APC. Exercising caution with APC in a patient with high-FiO2 requirements (risk of airway fire) is recommended.

Risk for airway fire is elevated in patients with FiO2 requirements greater than 40%, and thus cryotherapy is an advantageous technique for endoluminal obstructions. Cooling agents such as nitrous oxide and liquid nitrogen are used to repeatedly freeze and thaw tissue, ultimately rendering tissue nonviable. Also, the resistance of cartilage and fibrous tissue to thermal conductive effects of cryotherapy accounts for its safety. Efficacy has been shown for reduction in bleeding and hemoptysis [32]. Effects of cryotherapy, however, are temporary and delayed, and should not be used in an emergent CAO. Moreover, cryotherapy should not be utilized for extrinsic compression.

There is no role of photodynamic therapy in emergent CAO management.

4.4. Airway stenting

There are various materials and manufacturers of airway stents. Silicone stenting after an initial ablative procedure has been shown to safely maintain airway patency [33]. It is preferred over traditional metal stents that are commonly associated with airway perforation, granulation tissue formation, and bleeding. Popularly used and commonly known as the Dumon™ stent (Novatech), named after Jean Francois Dumon, it is a studded silicone stent that comes in a straight and Y-shaped mold (for saddling on carinal placement). The length and caliber of the stent is determined periprocedurally and is sized by the operant. Although stents are relatively thermoresistant and inexpensive, they do have the potential to migrate. Combined silicone and metal stents, known as hybrid stents, are frequently used but are more expensive. They combine the benefits of silicone and metal to give optimal compressive resistance while minimizing granulation tissue and perforation.

Another variant, the radioopaque Polyflex silicone stent (Boston Scientific) has synthetic threads that allow for stent flexibility and optimal thinness. These stents, however, have a greater risk of stent migration than the studded Dumon stent [34]. Finally, Dynamic Y stents are more anatomically forgiving, as they have anterior rings that mimic the tracheal lumen but the long length can impair mucous clearance. Overall, safety is high for these therapeutic interventions and complications such as pneumothorax, airway trauma, infection, stent migration, respiratory compromise, and death are low [35].

5. Postobstructive Pneumonia

Despite the paucity of literature outlining the management of postobstructive pneumonia, it is quite frequent in those with bronchogenic carcinoma. Most typically seen with small cell and squamous cell carcinomas, it can be caused by endobronchial involvement by a tumor or through extrinsic compression and parenchymal involvement. Other malignant causes include metastatic colon, breast, and renal cancers. Diagnosis is crucial as one must consider that the mortality of pneumonia is worse in those with underlying malignancy. Prolonged postobstructive pneumonia may lead to cavitation and necrosis. The intensivist should have a high degree of suspicion for postobstructive pneumonia in patients with radiographic evidence of atelectasis or mucous plugging. Diagnosis should be established and luminal patency should be estimated via CT imaging or endobronchial ultrasound (EBUS).

Patients with postobstructive pneumonia tend to have a longer duration of pulmonary symptoms, compared to those with uncomplicated community-acquired pneumonia. Also, rises in serum biomarkers such as the white blood cell count and procalcitonin are frequently not be observed. Those presenting with fever, however, have shown to provide greater bacteriologic yield [36–38]. Mortality, however, is higher [39].

Patients may present with signs and symptoms of septic shock (e.g., hypotension and tachycardia) or can be as uncomplicated as cough or dyspnea. Prior to any intervention, early antibiotic coverage must be initiated with appropriate coverage for Gram negative bacilli (*Enterobacter cloacae, Aacinetobacter sp*, and *Pseudomonas aeruginosa*), respiratory anaerobes, *Staphylococcus aureus* [40]. Patients can also be iatrogenically inoculated through interventional procedures, such as airway stent placement. The virulence of the inoculum is unclear; however, they may contribute to impaired innate airway mucous clearance.

The microbiota of postobstructive pneumonia appears to be polymicrobial and isolating an organism can be difficult. If microbiologic speciation is critical or if infection must be differentiated from alternative pathologic process, bronchoscopic sampling has greater yield than sputum culture [41]. Tumor debulking and airway reestablishment through interventional bronchoscopic techniques (argon plasma anticoagulation) help reduce mass effect and facilitate antibiotic penetration. Although it was studied as a palliative form of tumor burden, de Aquino Gorayeb et al. were able to demonstrate an improvement in performance status and postobstructive pneumonia (80% response) to high-dose brachytherapy [42].

If radiographic imaging is unavailable, intraprocedural empiric treatment should be considered, prior to therapeutic aspiration. Additionally, decanting pus from one airway still may provide a very brisk systemic response that must be treated aggressively with clinically appropriate volume resuscitation, in addition to aforementioned antibiotics. Antibiotic timeline must be tailored to the appropriate organism. The trachea, bronchus, and pulmonary

http://dx.doi.org/10.5772/65082

parenchyma provide a wide array of complications during the care of an oncologically critically ill patient. A judicious, yet timely systematic approach will ensure that the above aforementioned complications can be quickly dealt with.

6. Approach to Pneumothorax

Pneumothorax is defined as air in the pleural space. A common condition observed in the patients with malignancy and is more attributable to primary lesions than metastatic disease [43]. Pneumothorax can complicate an already deteriorating patient that may have subtle findings or can potentially require emergent intervention.

Traumatic
Blunt force
Iatrogenic
Thoracic surgery
Central venous catheter insertion
Transthoracic biopsy
Mechanical ventilation
Spontaneous
Primary
Secondary
Neoplastic (primary or metastatic)
Infectious
Interstitial lung disease (idiopathic, medication induced, radiation induced)
Chronic obstructive pulmonary disease
Cystic fibrosis [45]

Table 2. Classification of pneumothorax.

Here, we classify pneumothorax into primary spontaneous pneumothorax (PSP), secondary spontaneous pneumothorax (SSP), and traumatic pneumothorax. PSP occurs in patients without underlying lung disease. Secondary spontaneous pneumothorax is attributable to an underlying pulmonary disorder. Traumatic pneumothorax can be due to blunt physical trauma or from iatrogenic causes, such as invasive procedures and radiation therapy. Secondary spontaneous pneumothorax has shown an association with higher morbidity and mortality than primary spontaneous pneumothorax [44] (**Table 2**).

Iatrogenic pneumothorax is most common in hospitalized patients. Increasing incidence has correlated with the incidence of invasive diagnostic and therapeutic procedures, such as transthoracic lung biopsy and central venous catheter (CVC) insertion. Transthoracic needle aspiration is responsible for 45.7% and CVC in 24.8% [46]. Image guidance with CT for transthoracic biopsy reduced rates to 20% [47], although rates can vary significantly by institution. Currently, there is conflicting data whether smaller lesions or those with longer anatomic depth are associated with higher rates of pneumothorax [48]. As a complication of mechanical ventilation, pneumothorax carries an increase in morbidity and mortality, and has the highest risk of pneumothorax in the intensive care unit (ICU), particularly with the use of positive-end expiratory pressure [49, 50]. Rates of barotrauma have been noted to be as high as 15% [51].

Secondary spontaneous pneumothorax (SSP) is seen in both primary and metastatic diseases, regardless of pleural invasion. Tumor pleural involvement can cause cavitation, necrosis, and subsequent pleural damage. There have been many reports of pneumothorax secondary to chemotherapy administration [52–54] likely as a consequence of lysis of chemosensitive lesions.

Tension pneumothorax, as seen with mechanical ventilation or cardiopulmonary resuscitation, is a medical emergency. The incidence has not been definitively established, and statistical analysis is in its infancy [55]. Reports in adult ICUs have been as high as 3% [56]. Suspicion for such should be high when there is patient decompensation after known pneumothorax. It is suggested that delaying intervention until radiography has contributed to mortality [57]. This is a medical emergency and requires immediate mechanical decompression even before confirmation with imaging [58].

Bronchopleural fistula (BPF) is the presence of a significant, persistent air leakage after tube thoracostomy. Incidence has been reported up to 4.5% [59]. Occurrence of BPF has been reduced in recent years due to management of patients at risk (e.g., acute respiratory distress syndrome) with low tidal volume ventilation protocols [60, 61]. Despite this, knowledge of BPF is necessary for patients with a persistent pneumothorax and/or status post lung resection.

The mechanism involves airway disruption or alveolar rupture and can be due to mechanical volume overdistension [62, 63], elevated transpulmonary pressures [64], pleural trauma from an invasive procedure, or spontaneous rupture. Additional causes include inappropriate right main bronchus intubation and severe sepsis. Animal studies have demonstrated that excessive volume, rather than elevated airway pressures have been linked to alveolar rupture. Hence the term *volutrauma*, as opposed to *barotrauma*, more appropriately describes alveolar rupture [63]. Nevertheless, elevated transpulmonary pressures can play a major role in alveolar rupture [64]. Current recommendations, further outlined under *Management*, involve low-volume ventilation (≤6 mL/kg of predicted body weight), close monitoring for auto-PEEP, and avoidance of excessive hyperventilation [61].

6.1. Pathophysiology

In a normal lung, negative intrapleural pressure throughout the entire breathing cycle is maintained in the pleural space relative to the atmosphere, allowing for physiologic lung expansion, known as elastic recoil [65]. Transpulmonary pressure between lung alveoli and the pleura is disrupted due to alveolar permeability. This results in permeation of alveolar gas into low-resistance anatomic surfaces, such as the mediastinum, peritoneum, and pleural space. On inspiration, air that has translocated from alveoli enters directly to pleural cavity [66].

In tension physiology, once the nidus has occurred, the pleural cavity pressure equalizes with the chest wall environment causing a reduction of transpulmonary pressure, reducing vital capacity [67]. In the healthy awake adult, compensatory intrapleural pressures rise in attempt to compensate for tension pneumothorax. There is significant impairment of this with patients on mechanical ventilation, who usually are sedated. With positive pressure ventilation, inspiratory pressures are significantly elevated, creating an exaggerated pressure gradient. This is worsened from environmental air compressing lung parenchyma and distorting intrapleural pressure, risking mediastinal shift to the opposite lung and diaphragmatic depression. Alveoli may leak air into the pleura during inspiration only, creating a one-way valve effect, causing accumulation of pleural air. Rising pleural pressure can progress to affect nearby structures, resulting in ipsilateral lung deflation, mediastinal shift, and a rapid reduction in cardiac output [67].

6.2. Measurement

Assessing the size of a pneumothorax guides practitioners as to pursuing conservative versus invasive management. Light's index [68, 69] measures the percentile of pneumothorax:

Light's index = 100% − (diameter of collapsed lung^3/diameter of hemithorax^3) (100%). Light's index is helpful for quantifying reexpansion of lung after intervention [68, 69].

An alternative method involves measuring the average of the intrapleural distance at the level of the apical, mid-thorax, and basal levels. According to the British Medical Society, a "large" pneumothorax is defined as having >2 cm lung margin from the chest wall on roentgenogram [49]. Those classified as large warrants surgical decompression. It is important to note, however, that clinical symptoms outweigh measurement indices on interventional decision making.

6.3. Physical examination

Patients that develop secondary spontaneous pneumothorax present with varying degrees of severity dependent on the rate and volume of air accumulation, patient's age, status of mechanical ventilation, and baseline pulmonary function at the time of diagnosis. Because the pathophysiology involves a reduction in vital capacity, a predisposed lung can be presented with dramatic constellation of symptoms. Dyspnea, anxiety, and chest discomfort are common presenting symptoms [70]. Physical exam findings can include diminished breath sounds, increased manual percussion resonance on the ipsilateral affected lung, subcutaneous emphysema (Hamman's sign) [71], and tracheal deviation. Clinical signs can include tachypnea, oxygen desaturation, and increased work of breathing.

For the mechanically ventilated, frequent signs of tension pneumothorax include an acute onset of elevated pulmonary pressures (both peak and plateau) and hypotension [72]. Diagnosis includes obtaining chest radiography, which is demonstrated with a pleural line that is absent in lung markings beyond the line. However, it may take over 24 h for evidence after insult. A deep sulcus sign may only be the only radiographic evidence of pneumothorax, when seen on a supine image. Air collects basally, as opposed to the lung apex, causing a deepening of the costophrenic angle [73]. Diaphragmatic inversion with tracheal deviation is suggestive, although not pathognomonic, of tension pneumothorax [72]. Even with anatomic deviation, appropriate diagnosis was missed approximately half the time [74].

6.4. Management

American College of Chest Physicians (ACCP) guidelines provide recommendations based on patient stability and size of pneumothorax. Supplemental O_2 should be considered universally [44, 75], with caution taken for patients with chronic obstructive pulmonary disease and a proclivity to retain carbon dioxide. Small, stable pneumothoraces may be conservatively observed with appropriate follow up. Large pneumothoraces require hospitalization and needle or tube decompression.

Supplemental oxygen improves the rate of pleural air resorption through reduction of arterial nitrogen content. Reduced arterial nitrogen content creates a larger pleural space gradient, thus accelerating resorption of pleural air [44, 76].

Drainage is usually indicated in most patients with secondary spontaneous pneumothorax [44]. To further extrapolate indications for drainage, those who have symptomatic "large" SSP (as outlined earlier), the risk of resolution is outweighed by progressive risk of pleural compromise, and thoracostomy is warranted [77]. Small SSP (<2 cm from chest wall) can be managed with small bore chest tube. Asymptomatic patients with <1 cm from chest wall pneumothoraces can be managed conservatively with supplemental oxygen and serial chest radiography. Tube thoracostomy, when compared to needle decompression, has shown greater rate of success [44]. If a needle aspiration yields greater than 2.5 L of air, chest tube is indicated due to suspected air leak. Intervention can be guided with sonographic or fluoroscopic imaging if necessary.

Chest tube should be connected to water seal device and may be connected to a one-way Heimlich valve or low suction to aid reexpansion of lung [44]. Chest tube thoracostomy was successful in 78.1% of cases, and was not dependent on tube size [46]. If air leak has resolved and the lung has re-expanded on radiograph at least 12 h after last documented leak, the chest tube can be clamped, and removed after approximately 24 h [75]. Long term stabilization and pneumothorax recurrence may warrant intervention for prevention (e.g., pleurodesis) [44].

Persistent air leakage after 4 days of bronchopleural fistula after tube thoracostomy favors intervention over expectant management for spontaneous closure [44, 75, 77]. If a patient is mechanically ventilated, it is recommended to reduce tidal volume and airway pressures as tolerated, if not already done so [56]. Reducing overdistention of alveoli and development of intrinsic peep helps reduce transpulmonary gradients. This is achieved through the following maneuvers: Increasing inspiratory to expiratory ratio (I:E) through inspiratory flow control, decreasing tidal volume to ≤6 mL/kg predicted body weight, and adjusting the amount of ventilator driven patient breaths.

Bronchoscopic maneuvers such as deployment of endobronchial stenting, bronchoscopic valves [78], coiling [79, 80], injection of sclerosant, or laser coagulation has been utilized with efficacy [81–85].

Possible interventions include video-assisted thoracoscopic surgery (VATS) with mechanical or chemical pleurodesis, or VATS with resection of blebs. Additional chest tube placement or bronchoscopic intervention with the intent of sealing air leak is not recommended [75]. Chemical pleurodesis through tube thoracostomy is not recommended as well, although patients with poor surgical candidacy, current recommendations are talc slurry or doxycycline. Blood patch pleurodesis has shown outcomes with variable success [86, 87]. This is performed by instilling the patient's own venous blood (50-100 mL) into the pleural space through a chest tube.

Overall recurrence of secondary spontaneous pneumothorax is frequent [49]. We therefore recommend consideration for recurrence prevention through two options; surgical and chemical. Surgical options include VATS or open thoracotomy, depending on independent practitioner preference and patient candidacy. Open thoracotomy has shown lower recurrence rates but has higher blood loss and longer recovery times, and therefore, VATS with pleural obliteration is preferred [44, 75, 88]. Pleural obliteration can be achieved through pleurectomy, talc administration, and abrasion with gauze [89–91]. Chemical pleurodesis through tube thoracostomy has been shown to reduce recurrence of SSP, however success ranges 78–91% versus 95–100% with surgical intervention [44].

7. General Approach to Pleural Effusions

Approximately two-thirds of massive pleural effusions are associated with an underlying malignancy, [92] the majority of which present with 500–2000 mL of pleural fluid accumulation. Fluid collection can be serous, hematogenous, or serosanguinous. Of all exudative pleural effusions, pneumonia and malignancy are the two leading causes [93, 94]. In males, lung cancer is the most frequent metastatic pleural malignancy, breast cancer is most frequent in women [95, 96], and in up to 15% of cases, is unknown [97]. Often times recurrent, the responsible mechanism for pleural fluid accumulation is due to hilar and mediastinal lymphatic obstruction or seeding [92, 98]. Isolation of malignant cells in pleural fluid indicates a malignant pleural effusion (MPE). The development of hemothorax is due to the role of tumor angiogenesis, tumor invasion into blood vessels, or direct humoral capillary permeability [99]. Malignant pleural effusion (MPE) is a frequent complication of advanced malignancy, and carries a poor prognosis, affecting more than 150,000 people annually in the U.S. [100]. Median survival, depending on underlying malignancy, is less than 6 months once a diagnosis of MPE is made [96, 100]. MPE is diagnosed with malignant cells found in pleural fluid, which is often difficult to obtain. Pleural fluid analysis, in conjunction with the clinical history, is also sufficient to substantiate a diagnosis. Although in the ongoing years, the Light's criteria has faced scrutiny for excluding additional biomarkers (e.g., amylase) and including the closely correlated serum and pleural fluid lactate dehydrogenase (LDH) [101], it remains the mainstay of differentiating a transudative versus an exudative pleural effusion.

Light's criteria deems a pleural fluid as exudative if at least one of the following criteria are met [102]:

Pleural fluid protein/serum protein ratio greater than 0.5,

Pleural fluid LDH/serum LDH ratio greater than 0.6, or

Pleural fluid LDH greater than two-thirds the upper limits of the laboratory's normal serum LDH.

Amylase-rich pleural fluid can be suggestive of acute pancreatitis, esophageal rupture, or malignancy [103]. Recent studies have suggested that elevated serum lactate dehydrogenase to pleural fluid adenosine deaminase has been predictive of malignancy [104].

It is important to note, however, alternative causes of large pleural effusions in the setting of malignancy, such as congestive heart failure, venous thromboembolism, toxic effects of chemotherapy administration [105], radiation [106], low protein states, and pneumonia. Cytologic analysis of pleural fluid helps differentiate the underlying cause. Obstruction of the thoracic duct may also cause chylothorax and is suggested by pleural fluid triglyceride levels above 110 mg/dL (**Table 3**) [107].

Straw – Transudative process
Pus – Empyema
Red – Hemothorax
Pulmonary infarction
Postcardiac arrest
Iatrogenic (post procedure)
White – Chylothorax
Black – Aspergillosis
Ammonia – Urinothorax

Table 3. Qualitative description of pleural fluid.

Complicated parapneumonic effusions are often culture negative, have poor response to systemic antimicrobials, and may be loculated. Diagnosis is through pleural fluid analysis and utilization of the following criteria: pleural fluid pH less than 7.20, glucose level less than 60 mg/dL, and LDH > 1000 IU/L [108]. Meeting the aforementioned criterion renders a poor prognosis [109]. Complicated parapneumonic effusions warrant chest tube placement that otherwise runs the risk of progression to thoracic empyema [110]. The majority of organisms isolated through fluid culture or Gram stain consist of staphylococci and anaerobes such as *Fusobacterium, Peptostreptococcus, Bacteroides fragilis,* and *Prevotella* species [111, 112]. Long-term sequelae of unresolving empyema, hemothorax, and surgical manipulation may result in a trapped lung. Trapped lung occurs when reexpansion of atelectatic lung is impaired due to a fibrinous peel overlying visceral pleura, creating a chronic pleural effusion. Lung entrapment, in turn, is an unexpandable lung due to active malignancy or infection [113, 114]. For patients with significantly trapped lung, pleurodesis can be deferred.

Chemotherapy associated with large-volume effusions include methotrexate, procarbazine, cyclophosphamide, mitomycin, bleomycin, and IL-1 (**Table 4**) [106].

Malignancies associated with malignant pleural effusions [62]	Indirect causes of pleural effusions (paramalignant)
Lung 37.5%	Local tumor effect
Breast 16.8%	Trapped lung
Lymphoma 11.5%	Chylothorax
Genitourinary 9.4%	Lymphatic obstruction
GI tract 6.8%	SVC (superior vena cava) syndrome
	Pulmonary embolism
	Hypoalbuminemic state
	Chemotherapy/radiation therapy (incomplete)
	Tumor necrosis factor
	Interleukin-2
	Methotrexate
	Bleomycin
	Cyclophosphamide

Table 4. Malignant and indirect (paramalignant) causes of effusions.

Severity in symptoms is dependent on residual lung function, acuity in rate of fluid accumulation, and whether or not the patient is on mechanical ventilation. Large pleural effusions are often symptomatic and results in reduced chest wall compliance and lung volume [115]. These include orthopnea, cough, dyspnea, and fever. Examination of the affected lung may include diminished breath sounds, tactile fremitus, and crackles. Tracheal deviation may also be a presenting finding with larger-volume effusions. Diagnosis of pleural effusion is suspected with physical examination and confirmed radiographically. Treatment can be either palliative or aimed at improving survival. Reaccumulation of MPE can worsen a patient's symptoms; however, in asymptomatic individuals, cost, preference, and functional status should be taken into account.

Diagnostic and therapeutic considerations with large volumes are first achieved with thoracentesis [116]. Pleural fluid analysis helps determine between transudative or exudative effusions and may indicate the primary cause [117]. The severity of symptoms and global prognosis of the patient dictates the necessity of further invasiveness [118]. Recurrence is high with therapeutic aspiration without pleurodesis incurs a high rate. Thoracentesis is not without complications, including pneumothorax, empyema, and adhesions [96]. Other procedures include pleural biopsy, bronchoscopy, pleuroscopy, and video-assisted thoracoscopic surgery (VATS) with biopsy.

In the setting of clinical acuity, such as hemodynamic compromise, tracheal deviation, diminishing hypoxemia, or a progressively unstable airway, emergent indication is indicated for lung reexpansion. Thoracentesis should be performed for relief of symptoms, and chest tube drainage is recommended for empyema and/or complicated parapneumonic effusions. If a patient has a very limited lifespan (i.e., <1 month), pleurodesis is less strongly recommended. Aspiration on each occasion should not exceed 1.5 L to avoid reexpansion of pulmonary edema [119].

Inadequate or improperly draining tubes may warrant decortication. Nearly all patients with malignant pleural effusion who undergo drainage face recurrence within 30 days [120, 121]. Such patients benefit from pleurodesis, when in consideration of life expectancy. Repeat thoracentesis is selectively recommended for patients with short life expectancy, as it can lead to formation of adhesions, mentioned earlier. Repeat aspiration helps palliate symptoms for the terminally ill, especially with the use of small-bore catheters [122].

Pleurodesis can be done surgically or chemically. Chemical pleurodesis may require a prolonged hospital stay and carries a small risk of pneumonitis [123]. Thoracoscopic pleurodesis is recommended over catheter based [124, 125].

Surgical outcomes are often difficult to achieve due to poor surgical candidacy. Chemical pleurodesis involves infusion of a sclerosing agent such as talc (poudrage or slurry), 5-FU, minocycline, bleomycin, and silver nitrate, with talc being the most successful agent for providing reaccumulation after 1 month [126–128].

Pleurodesis helps achieve lung expansion and reestablishes normal symphysis of visceral and parietal pleura. The primary mechanism involves inciting a broad spread inflammatory response, in turn promoting fibrin deposits [129]. Suspected antitumor effects of talc by induction of apoptosis of cancer cells may also help provide a role in blunting tumor progression intrapleurally. Bleomycin carries a well-established antineoplastic role [130]. With recent meta-analyses, both talc poudrage and slurry are equally efficacious with thoracoscopic technique considered ideal [96].

Alternatives include chronic indwelling catheter placement, which is an increasingly popular option due to its low risk of infection, displacement, and manageability as an outpatient [131].

Both talc pleurodesis and chronic indwelling catheters have been shown to be effective initial treatments for MPE [126]. Indwelling catheters also have a role once a patient develops trapped lung.

For clinically stable patients with poor response to initial thoracostomy drainage or with multiloculated effusions, and are poor candidates for surgical intervention, intrapleural tissue plasminogen activator (tPA) combined with DNase has been a growingly influential therapy, without additional excess of adverse events [132, 133]. Administration of fibrinolytics or DNase alone did not improve outcomes [133, 134]. Pleuroperitoneal shunting is an additional option to consider, especially in patients with trapped lung (**Table 5**) [100, 109].

Thoracentesis/ thoracostomy	Large pleural effusions. Thoracostomy for chest tube insertion, fibrinolysis, and pleurodesis.
Pleurodesis	Recurrent pleural effusion
Video-assisted thoracoscopic surgery (VATS)	Complicated/parapneumonic effusion, pleurodesis, and pleurectomy. Lysis of adhesions, blebectomy, decortication, lobectomy, and lung volume reduction. Contraindicated in hemodynamic instability. Less invasive and painful than thoracotomy.
Thoracotomy with decortication	Major surgery. Full mediastinal visualization. Better for large tumors, close to mediastinal/vascular structures. Higher risk of complications and estimated blood loss [101].
PleurX® catheter	Can be managed outpatient, role palliative care.
Pleuroperitoneal shunt	Exhaustion of alternative options, useful for chylothorax in managing nutritional and immunologic status.

Table 5. Interventional procedures in management of massive pleural effusion.

8. Approach to Hemothorax

Hemothorax is evident when frank blood is aspirated from pleural space during thoracentesis, tube thoracostomy, or VATS, and is confirmed when pleural fluid hematocrit exceeds more than >50% of serum hematocrit concentration. Pleural bleeding can be simplified as being due to mediastinal or pleural tissue insult. Diagnosis is mainly attributable to mechanical chest trauma, and its overall incidence has not been well quantified. Nontraumatic hemothorax is most commonly due to malignancy and is explained by the role of tumor angiogenesis, invasion into blood vessels, or direct humoral capillary permeability [99]. Not to be confused with a bloody tap, where the latter instance clears after centrifuge, hemothorax has a propensity to not clot due to continuing defibrination from mediastinal motion. Other causes may be a consequence of iatrogenic anticoagulation [136], pulmonary embolism causing pulmonary infarction, or catamenial hemothorax [137, 138]. Surgical manipulation, such as thoracentesis, bronchoscopic biopsy, mediastinoscopy [139], needle biopsy, and central venous catheter insertion may also be a cause [140]. Spontaneous hemothorax, i.e., hemothorax without identifiable cause, is infrequent [141]. Causes are outlined below (**Table 6**) [75].

Nontraumatic	
Neoplastic	
	Metastatic diseases
	Vascular malignancy
	Bronchogenic carcinoma
	Mesothelioma
	Angiosarcoma
Coagulopathy	
	Anticoagulation
	Thrombocytopenia
	Congenital disorders
Pulmonary embolism	
Pulmonary infarct	
Vascular	
	Arteriovenous malformation
	Aneurysm
	Connective tissue disease
	Aortic dissection
Traumatic	
Central venous catheter	
Thoracentesis	
Transbronchial biopsy	
Percutaneous needle aspirate	
Pleural biopsy	
Thoracic surgery	

Table 6. Nontraumatic and traumatic causes of hemorrhagic pleural effusions.

8.1. Imaging

Hemothorax and pleural effusion is not distinguishable on routine chest radiography or ultrasonography. Presenting history aids index of suspicion helps distinguishing between hemothorax and pleural effusion. Chest CT imaging blood presents with higher attenuation than pleural effusion. Later stages of hemothorax can include pleural deposition, thickening, and loculation [142]. CT imaging is also well associated with determining the necessity of VATS [143]. Hemopneumothorax is characterized by a pneumothorax with ipsilateral air-fluid level. Suspicion for vascular etiologies may warrant CT angiography.

8.2. Management

Outlining the management of a patient with confirmed hemothorax in the intensive care unit depends on patient stability and prognosis, and spans from supportive care to emergent thoracotomy [144]. Goals of care are for blood evacuation to avoid fibrin deposition and subsequent trapped lung, and the development of empyema [145].

Discontinuation of anticoagulant therapy and correction of any coagulopathy is recommended if hemothorax is attributable to systemic anticoagulation [145, 146]. Massive hemothorax may require blood transfusion resuscitation. Blood collection in the pleural space in minimal amounts may spontaneously reabsorb; however, chest tube drainage is necessary for rapidly developing hemothorax [27]. Drainage reestablishes parieto-pleural symphysis and creates a tamponade if the source of bleeding is from pleural rupture. With concomitant pneumothorax, i.e., hemopneumothorax, drainage is definitively indicated. In contrast to chest tube management of spontaneous pneumothorax, large-bore chest tubes should be placed due to the rapidity of clotting [75, 146, 147].

Thoracotomy is warranted for the hemodynamically unstable and those with massive hemothorax. This constitutes patients with severely rapid exsanguination with retained volume greater than 500 mL, accumulated output over 1500 mL, or if exsanguination is above 200 ml per h [139, 148]. Chest tubes can be maintained in the chest wall cavity until the amount of tube drainage in 24 h is less than 100 mL but removal should not be prolonged to reduce the risk of infectious inoculation [149]. Residual clotted blood after thoracostomy should be removed thoracoscopically to reduce the risk of empyema and fibrothorax [150]. Fibrothoraces that require VATS decortication should be delayed months after initial insult in order to allow coalescence and stabilization of a fibrin peel [145]. VATS permits safe decortication of adhesions and removal of clotted blood. The role of intrapleural fibrinolytics in the management of hemothorax is currently in its infancy. VATS has better proven efficacy and shorter Hospitalization stay [135]; however, fibrinolytics are a considerable option when patients are without underlying coagulopathy but are clinically unstable for VATS [148, 151–153]. Fibrinolytics can be applied for chemical lysis of intrapleural adhesions, commonly seen with fibrothorax [75]. There is no evidence indicating systemic side effects to intrapleural fibrinolysis. Antimicrobials early in the treatment of traumatic hemothorax reduce rates of empyema. There is evidence showing benefit in prophylactic administration spontaneous pneumothorax as well. Initial antibiotic coverage for empyema should include *Staphylococcus* and *Streptococcus* [154].

9. Conclusion

Substantial challenges present themselves in the ICU, with airway compromise being one of the high priorities. Either caused by primary cancers or secondary metastasis, the upper and lower airways have very little room for error. Hemorrhaging from or into the nasopharynx, trachea, and its tributaries can precipitate an inability to ventilate and oxygenate rapidly. Understanding the anatomical and physiological challenges are the first steps to managing such complex scenarios. Rapid stabilization with nasal packing and/or protection of ventilatory units, via intubation, is an essential task for the intensivist. Subsequently understanding or having a high index of suspicion as to the origin of respiratory failure helps prevent further decline in respiratory status. Central airway obstruction requires urgent/emergent advanced bronchoscopic evaluation with potential therapeutic intervention. One must be also cognizant that large pleural effusions (of varying origin) and/or pneumothoraces contribute to the spectrum of emergencies faced in an oncological critical care unit.

Author details

Osheen Abramian[1], Diana Kolman[2] and Emil Abramian[3*]

*Address all correspondence to: emil.abramian@ctca-hope.com

1 Internal Medicine, Drexel University College of Medicine, Philadelphia, USA

2 Interventional Pulmonology, Cooper University Hospital, Camden, USA

3 Interventional Pulmonology, Cancer Treatment Centers of America, Philadelphia, USA

References

[1] Delank, K.W., *Diagnosis and therapy of epistaxis*. Laryngorhinootologie, 2006. 85(8): pp. 593–603; quiz 604–608.

[2] Lopez, F., et al., Metastases to nasal cavity and paranasal sinuses. Head Neck, 2016. doi: 10.1002/hed.24502. [Epub ahead of print]

[3] Barnes, M.L., Spielmann, P.M. and White, P.S., *Epistaxis: a contemporary evidence based approach*. Otolaryngol Clin North Am, 2012. 45(5): pp. 1005–1017.

[4] Kucik, C.J. and Clenney, T., *Management of epistaxis*. Am Fam Physician, 2005. 71(2): pp. 305–311.

[5] McGarry, G.W., *Nasal endoscope in posterior epistaxis: a preliminary evaluation*. J Laryngol Otol, 1991. 105(6): pp. 428–431.

[6] Bertrand, B., et al., Guidelines to the management of epistaxis.B-ENT, 2005,1, Suppl. 1, 27-43

[7] Tanner, R. and Harney, M.S., *The initial management of epistaxis*. Ir Med J, 2015. 108(4): pp. 123–124.

[8] Williams, M. and Onslow, J., *Airway difficulties associated with severe epistaxis*. Anaesthesia, 1999. 54(8): pp. 812–813.

[9] Lin, Y.T. and Orkin, L.R., *Arterial hypoxemia in patients with anterior and posterior nasal packings*. Laryngoscope, 1979. 89(1): pp. 140–144.

[10] Melia, L. and McGarry, G.W., *Epistaxis: update on management*. Curr Opin Otolaryngol Head Neck Surg, 2011. 19(1): pp. 30–35.

[11] Amin, M., et al., *Silver nitrate cauterisation, does concentration matter?* Clin Otolaryngol, 2007. 32(3): pp. 197–199.

[12] Webb, B.D., et al., *Primary tracheal malignant neoplasms: the University of Texas MD Anderson Cancer Center experience*. J Am Coll Surg, 2006. 202(2): pp. 237–246.

[13] Ernst, A., et al., *Central airway obstruction*. Am J Respir Crit Care Med, 2004. 169(12): pp. 1278–1297.

[14] Cahill, B.C. and Ingbar, D.H., *Massive hemoptysis. Assessment and management*. Clin Chest Med, 1994. 15(1): pp. 147–167.

[15] Mason, R., etal., (2016). Murray and Nadel's Textbook of Respiratory Medicine (6th ed., Vol. 1 &2). Philadelphia, PA: Elsevier.

[16] Miller, R.R. and McGregor, D.H., *Hemorrhage from carcinoma of the lung*. Cancer, 1980. 46(1): pp. 200–205.

[17] Ibrahim, W.H., *Massive haemoptysis: the definition should be revised*. Eur Respir J, 2008. 32(4): pp. 1131–1132.

[18] Dweik, R.A. and Stoller, J.K., *Role of bronchoscopy in massive hemoptysis*. Clin Chest Med, 1999. 20(1): pp. 89–105.

[19] Jeudy, J., et al., *ACR Appropriateness Criteria hemoptysis*. J Thorac Imag, 2010. 25(3): pp. W67–69.

[20] Swanson, K.L., et al., *Bronchial artery embolization: experience with 54 patients*. Chest, 2002. 121(3): pp. 789–795.

[21] Sakr, L. and Dutau, H., *Massive hemoptysis: an update on the role of bronchoscopy in diagnosis and management*. Respiration, 2010. 80(1): pp. 38–58.

[22] Ernst, A., et al., *Principles and Practice of Interventional Pulmonology*. 1st Ed. Springer Science, New York 2013

[23] Pfleger, A. and Eber, E., *Assessment and causes of stridor*. Paediatr Respir Rev, 2016. 18: pp. 64–72.

[24] Terlinden, N., et al., *An innovative approach to tracheotomy in patients with major obstruction of the upper airway*. Am J Otolaryngol, 2014. 35(3): pp. 445–8.

[25] Chin, B.S., et al., *Emergency tracheostomy for advanced head and neck tumor*. J Surg Oncol, 1998. 67(1): pp. 49–51.

[26] Varghese, B.T., Balakrishnan, M. and Kuriakose, R., *Fibre-optic intubation in oncological head and neck emergencies*. J Laryngol Otol, 2005. 119(8): pp. 634–638.

[27] Delius, R.E., et al., *Catheter aspiration for simple pneumothorax. Experience with 114 patients*. Arch Surg, 1989. 124(7): pp. 833–836.

[28] Colt, H.G. and Harrell, J.H., *Therapeutic rigid bronchoscopy allows level of care changes in patients with acute respiratory failure from central airways obstruction*. Chest, 1997. 112(1): pp. 202–206.

[29] Ost, D.E., et al., *Therapeutic bronchoscopy for malignant central airway obstruction: success rates and impact on dyspnea and quality of life*. Chest, 2015. 147(5): pp. 1282–1298.

[30] Amjadi, K., et al., *Impact of interventional bronchoscopy on quality of life in malignant airway obstruction*. Respiration, 2008. 76(4): pp. 421–428.

[31] Boyd, M. and Rubio, E., *The utility of interventional pulmonary procedures in liberating patients with malignancy-associated central airway obstruction from mechanical ventilation*. Lung, 2012. 190(5): pp. 471–476.

[32] Marasso, A., et al., *Cryosurgery in bronchoscopic treatment of tracheobronchial stenosis. Indications, limits, personal experience*. Chest, 1993. 103(2): pp. 472–474.

[33] Dumon, J.F., *A dedicated tracheobronchial stent*. Chest, 1990. 97(2): pp. 328–332.

[34] Feller-Kopman, D., *Acute complications of artificial airways*. Clin Chest Med, 2003. 24(3): pp. 445–455.

[35] Ost, D.E., et al., *Complications following therapeutic bronchoscopy for malignant central airway obstruction: results of the AQuIRE registry*. Chest, 2015. 148(2): pp. 450–471.

[36] Liao, W.Y., et al., *Bacteriology of infected cavitating lung tumor*. Am J Respir Crit Care Med, 2000. 161(5): pp. 1750–1753.

[37] Semaan, R. and Yarmus, L., *Rigid bronchoscopy and silicone stents in the management of central airway obstruction*. J Thorac Dis, 2015. 7(Suppl 4): pp. S352–362.

[38] Hsu-Kim, C., et al., *The microbiology of postobstructive pneumonia in lung cancer patients*. J Bronchology Interv Pulmonol, 2013. 20(3): pp. 266–270.

[39] Abers, M.S., et al., *Postobstructive Pneumonia: an underdescribed syndrome*. Clin Infect Dis, 2016. 62(8): pp. 957–961.

[40] Frei III, E., et al., (2003) Holland Frei Cancer Medicine, (6th ed.) Hamilton (ON):BC Decker.

[41] Mehta, R.M. and Cutaia, M., *The role of interventional pulmonary procedures in the management of post-obstructive pneumonia*. Curr Infect Dis Rep, 2006. 8(3): pp. 207–214.

[42] de Aquino Gorayeb, M.M., et al., High-dose-rate brachytherapy in symptom palliation due to malignant endobronchial obstruction: a quantitative assessment. Brachytherapy, 2013,12(5): pp.471–478

[43] Chen, C.H., et al., *Secondary spontaneous pneumothorax: which associated conditions benefit from pigtail catheter treatment?* Am J Emerg Med, 2012. 30(1): pp. 45–50.

[44] MacDuff, A., et al., *Management of spontaneous pneumothorax: British Thoracic Society Pleural Disease Guideline 2010*. Thorax, 2010. 65(Suppl. 2): pp. ii18–31.

[45] Flume, P.A., et al., *Pneumothorax in cystic fibrosis*. Chest, 2005. 128(2): pp. 720–728.

[46] Noh, T.O. and Ryu, K.M., *Comparative study for the efficacy of small bore catheter in the patients with iatrogenic pneumothorax*. Korean J Thorac Cardiovasc Surg, 2011. 44(6): pp. 418–22.

[47] McSweeney, S.E., et al., *Evaluation of the efficacy and safety of percutaneous biopsy of lung*. Open Respir Med J, 2012. 6: pp. 82–88.

[48] Geraghty, P.R., et al., *CT-guided transthoracic needle aspiration biopsy of pulmonary nodules: needle size and pneumothorax rate*. Radiology, 2003. 229(2): pp. 475–481.

[49] Gammon, R.B., Shin, M.S. and Buchalter, S.E., *Pulmonary barotrauma in mechanical ventilation. Patterns and risk factors*. Chest, 1992. 102(2): pp. 568–572.

[50] de Lassence, A., et al., *Pneumothorax in the intensive care unit: incidence, risk factors, and outcome*. Anesthesiology, 2006. 104(1): pp. 5–13.

[51] Strange, C., *Pleural complications in the intensive care unit*. Clin Chest Med, 1999. 20(2): pp. 317–27.

[52] Gennatas, S., et al., *Early pneumothorax as a feature of response to crizotinib therapy in a patient with ALK rearranged lung adenocarcinoma*. BMC Cancer, 2013. 13: 207 p.

[53] Ahmed, M.S., *Spontaneous bilateral pneumothorax in a patient with metastatic synovial sarcoma while under chemotherapy*. Transl Lung Cancer Res, 2012. 1(4): pp. 289–291.

[54] Chen, J.R. and Yang, Y.C., *Spontaneous pneumothorax after intensive chemotherapy in endometrial cancer: a rare complication*. Taiwan J Obstet Gynecol, 2014. 53(2): pp. 245–247.

[55] Roberts, D.J., et al., *Clinical manifestations of tension pneumothorax: protocol for a systematic review and meta-analysis*. Syst Rev, 2014. 3: 3 p.

[56] Litmanovitch, M., et al., *Persistent bronchopleural fistula in a patient with adult respiratory distress syndrome. Treatment with pressure-controlled ventilation*. Chest, 1993. 104(6): pp. 1901–1902.

[57] Steier, M., et al., *Pneumothorax complicating continuous ventilatory support*. J Thorac Cardiovasc Surg, 1974. 67(1): pp. 17–23.

[58] Light, R.W., *Tension pneumothorax*. Intensive Care Med, 1994. 20(7): pp. 468–469.

[59] Sirbu, H., et al., *Bronchopleural fistula in the surgery of non-small cell lung cancer: incidence, risk factors, and management*. Ann Thorac Cardiovasc Surg, 2001. 7(6): pp. 330–336.

[60] Kempainen, R.R. and Pierson, D.J., *Persistent air leaks in patients receiving mechanical ventilation*. Semin Respir Crit Care Med, 2001. 22(6): pp. 675–684.

[61] Luks, A.M. and Pierson, D.J., *Barotrauma and bronchopleural fistula*. In: Principles and Practice of Mechanical Ventilation. 23rd ed, Tobin, M.J. (ed.). New York: McGraw-Hill, 2012. 44: pp1041-1063.

[62] Dreyfuss, D., et al., *High inflation pressure pulmonary edema. Respective effects of high airway pressure, high tidal volume, and positive end-expiratory pressure*. Am Rev Respir Dis, 1988. 137(5): pp. 1159–1164.

[63] Dreyfuss, D. and Saumon, G., *Barotrauma is volutrauma, but which volume is the one responsible?* Intensive Care Med, 1992. 18(3): pp. 139–1341.

[64] Doelken P and Sahn, S., *Pleural disease in the critically ill patient*. In: Intensive Care Medicine. 6th ed, Irwin, R.S., Rippe, J.M. (eds.). Philadelphia: Lippincott Williams and Wilkins, 2008: pp 686.

[65] Norris, R.M., Jones, J.G. and Bishop, J.M., *Respiratory gas exchange in patients with spontaneous pneumothorax*. Thorax, 1968. 23(4): pp. 427–433.

[66] Choi, W.I., *Pneumothorax*. Tuberc Respir Dis (Seoul), 2014. 76(3): pp. 99–104.

[67] Rutherford, R.B., et al., *The pathophysiology of progressive, tension pneumothorax*. J Trauma, 1968. 8(2): pp. 212–227.

[68] Light, R.W., *Pleural Diseases: Pneumothorax*. 3rd ed. Baltimore: Williams and Wilkins, 1990.

[69] Noppen, M., et al., *Quantification of the size of primary spontaneous pneumothorax: accuracy of the Light index*. Respiration, 2001. 68(4): pp. 396–399.

[70] Dines, D.E., Clagett, O.T. and Payne, W.S., *Spontaneous pneumothorax in emphysema*. Mayo Clin Proc, 1970. 45(7): pp. 481–487.

[71] Sarkar, M., et al., *Auscultation of the respiratory system*. Ann Thorac Med, 2015. 10(3): pp. 158–168.

[72] Leigh-Smith, S. and Harris, T., *Tension pneumothorax—time for a re-think?* Emerg Med J, 2005. 22(1): pp. 8–16.

[73] Matsumoto, S., et al., *Diagnostic accuracy of oblique chest radiograph for occult pneumothorax: comparison with ultrasonography*. World J Emerg Surg, 2016. 11: 5 p.

[74] Spiteri, M.A., Cook, D.G. and Clarke, S.W., *Reliability of eliciting physical signs in examination of the chest*. Lancet, 1988. 1(8590): pp. 873–875.

[75] Baumann, M.H., et al., *Management of spontaneous pneumothorax: an American College of Chest Physicians Delphi consensus statement*. Chest, 2001. 119(2): pp. 590–602.

[76] Northfield, T.C., *Oxygen therapy for spontaneous pneumothorax*. Br Med J, 1971. 4(5779): pp. 86–88.

[77] Schoenenberger, R.A., et al., *Timing of invasive procedures in therapy for primary and secondary spontaneous pneumothorax*. Arch Surg, 1991. 126(6): pp. 764–766.

[78] Mahajan, A.K., Doeing, D.C. and Hogarth, D.K., *Isolation of persistent air leaks and placement of intrabronchial valves*. J Thorac Cardiovasc Surg, 2013. 145(3): pp. 626–630.

[79] Sivrikoz, C.M., et al., *Effective approach for the treatment of bronchopleural fistula: application of endovascular metallic ring-shaped coil in combination with fibrin glue*. Ann Thorac Surg, 2007. 83(6): pp. 2199–2201.

[80] Watanabe, S., Watanabe, T. and Urayama, H., *Endobronchial occlusion method of bronchopleural fistula with metallic coils and glue*. Thorac Cardiovasc Surg, 2003. 51(2): pp. 106–108.

[81] Takahashi, M., et al., *Ultraflex expandable stents for the management of air leaks*. Ann Thorac Cardiovasc Surg, 2006. 12(1): pp. 50–52.

[82] Bellato, V., et al., *Management of postoperative bronchopleural fistula with a tracheobronchial stent in a patient requiring mechanical ventilation*. Intensive Care Med, 2010. 36(4): pp. 721–722.

[83] Martin, W.R., Siefkin, A.D. and Allen, R., *Closure of a bronchopleural fistula with bronchoscopic instillation of tetracycline*. Chest, 1991. 99(4): pp. 1040–1042.

[84] Wang, K.P., et al., *NdYAG laser closure of a bronchopleural fistula*. Monaldi Arch Chest Dis, 1993. 48(4): pp. 301–303.

[85] Akulian, J. and Feller-Kopman, D., *The past, current and future of diagnosis and management of pleural disease*. J Thorac Dis, 2015. 7(Suppl. 4): pp. S329–338.

[86] Cagirici, U., et al., *Autologous blood patch pleurodesis in spontaneous pneumothorax with persistent air leak*. Scand Cardiovasc J, 1998. 32(2): pp. 75–78.

[87] Kelly, M.G., *Acute respiratory distress syndrome (ARDS) secondary to talc pleurodesis*. Eur J Intern Med, 2007. 18(8): 611 p.

[88] Light, R.W., *Pleural Diseases*. 6th ed. Philadelphia: Williams and Wilkins, 2013.

[89] Fosse, E., et al., *Thoracoscopic pleurodesis*. Scand J Thorac Cardiovasc Surg, 1993. 27(3–4): pp. 117–119.

[90] Milanez, J.R., et al., *Intrapleural talc for the prevention of recurrent pneumothorax*. Chest, 1994. 106(4): pp. 1162–1165.

[91] Bobbio, A., et al., *Thoracoscopic parietal pleural argon beam coagulation versus pleural abrasion in the treatment of primary spontaneous pneumothorax*. Eur J Cardiothorac Surg, 2006. 29(1): pp. 6–8.

[92] Chernow, B. and Sahn, S.A., *Carcinomatous involvement of the pleura: an analysis of 96 patients*. Am J Med, 1977. 63(5): pp. 695–702.

[93] Assi, Z., et al., *Cytologically proved malignant pleural effusions: distribution of transudates and exudates*. Chest, 1998. 113(5): pp. 1302–1304.

[94] Ashchi, M., et al., *Transudative malignant pleural effusions: prevalence and mechanisms*. South Med J, 1998. 91(1): pp. 23–26.

[95] Light, R.W., *Management of pleural effusions*. J Formos Med Assoc, 2000. 99(7): pp. 523–531.

[96] Roberts, M.E., et al., *Management of a malignant pleural effusion: British Thoracic Society Pleural Disease Guideline 2010*. Thorax, 2010. 65(Suppl. 2): pp. ii32–40.

[97] Johnston, W.W., *The malignant pleural effusion. A review of cytopathologic diagnoses of 584 specimens from 472 consecutive patients*. Cancer, 1985. 56(4): pp. 905–909.

[98] Agrawal, A., et al., *Clinico- pathological profile and course of malignant pleural effusion in a tertiary care teaching hospital in western U.P. with special reference to lung cancer*. Lung India, 2015. 32(4): pp. 326–330.

[99] Kanou, S., et al., *A case of hepatocellular carcinoma with direct invasion into the pleural cavity presenting as hemorrhage achieved hemostasis with intra-arterial injection of ethanol*. Nihon Shokakibyo Gakkai Zasshi, 1996. 93(10): pp. 753–757.

[100] *American Thoracic Society, Management of malignant pleural effusions*. Am J Respir Crit Care Med, 2000. 162(5): pp. 1987–2001.

[101] Heffner, J.E., Brown, L.K. and Barbieri, C.A., *Diagnostic value of tests that discriminate between exudative and transudative pleural effusions. Primary Study Investigators*. Chest, 1997. 111(4): pp. 970–980.

[102] Light, R.W., et al., *Pleural effusions: the diagnostic separation of transudates and exudates*. Ann Intern Med, 1972. 77(4): pp. 507–513.

[103] Joseph, J., et al., *A prospective study of amylase-rich pleural effusions with special reference to amylase isoenzyme analysis*. Chest, 1992. 102(5): pp. 1455–1459.

[104] Verma, A., Abisheganaden, J. and Light, R.W., *Identifying malignant pleural effusion by a cancer ratio (Serum LDH: pleural fluid ADA ratio)*. Lung, 2016. 194(1): pp. 147–153.

[105] Libshitz, H.I., *Radiation changes in the lung*. Semin Roentgenol, 1993. 28(4): pp. 303–320.

[106] Morelock, S.Y. and Sahn, S.A., *Drugs and the pleura*. Chest, 1999. 116(1): pp. 212–221.

[107] Maldonado, F., et al., *Pleural fluid characteristics of chylothorax*. Mayo Clin Proc, 2009. 84(2): pp. 129–133.

[108] Light, R.W., et al., *Parapneumonic effusions*. Am J Med, 1980. 69(4): pp. 507–512.

[109] R.W. (ed.). Philadelphia: Lippincott Williams and Wilkins, 2013. Pp133-161

[110] Mavroudis, C., et al., *Experimental aerobic-anaerobic thoracic empyema in the guinea pig*. Ann Thorac Surg, 1987. 43(3): pp. 298–302.

[111] Brook, I. and Frazier, E.H., *Aerobic and anaerobic microbiology of empyema. A retrospective review in two military hospitals*. Chest, 1993. 103(5): pp. 1502–1507.

[112] Bartlett, J.G., et al., *Bacteriology of empyema*. Lancet, 1974. 1(7853): pp. 338–340.

[113] Doelken, P., *Clinical implications of unexpandable lung due to pleural disease*. Am J Med Sci, 2008. 335(1): pp. 21–25.

[114] Huggins, J.T., Doelken, P. and Sahn, S.A., *The unexpandable lung*. F1000 Med Rep, 2010. 2: 77 p.

[115] Judson M and Sahn, S., *Pulmonary physiologic abnormalities caused by pleural disease*. Semin Respir Crit Care Med, 1995. 16: pp. 346–353.

[116] Light, R.W., *Clinical practice. Pleural effusion*. N Engl J Med, 2002. 346(25): pp. 1971–1977.

[117] Light, R.W., Erozan, Y.S. and Ball Jr., W.C., *Cells in pleural fluid. Their value in differential diagnosis*. Arch Intern Med, 1973. 132(6): pp. 854–860.

[118] Antony, V.B., et al., *Management of malignant pleural effusions*. Eur Respir J, 2001. 18(2): pp. 402–419.

[119] Mahfood, S., et al., *Reexpansion pulmonary edema*. Ann Thorac Surg, 1988. 45(3): pp. 340–345.

[120] Viallat, J.R., et al., *Thoracoscopic talc poudrage pleurodesis for malignant effusions. A review of 360 cases*. Chest, 1996. 110(6): pp. 1387–1393.

[121] Sarna, L., et al., *Quality of life and meaning of illness of women with lung cancer*. Oncol Nurs Forum, 2005. 32(1): pp. E9–19.

[122] Parulekar, W., et al., *Use of small-bore vs large-bore chest tubes for treatment of malignant pleural effusions*. Chest, 2001. 120(1): pp. 19–25.

[123] Kennedy, L., et al., *Pleurodesis using talc slurry*. Chest, 1994. 106(2): pp. 342–346.

[124] Kvale, P.A., et al., *Palliative care in lung cancer: ACCP evidence-based clinical practice guidelines (2nd ed)*. Chest, 2007. 132(Suppl. 3): pp. 368S–403S.

[125] Shaw, P. and Agarwal, R., *Pleurodesis for malignant pleural effusions*. Cochrane DB Syst Rev, 2004. (1): CD002916

[126] Xia, H., et al., *Efficacy and safety of talc pleurodesis for malignant pleural effusion: a meta-analysis*. PLoS One, 2014. 9(1): e87060 p.

[127] Diacon, A.H., et al., *Prospective randomized comparison of thoracoscopic talc poudrage under local anesthesia versus bleomycin instillation for pleurodesis in malignant pleural effusions*. Am J Respir Crit Care Med, 2000. 162(4 Pt 1): pp. 1445–1449.

[128] Kuzdzal, J., et al., *Talc powder vs doxycycline in the control of malignant pleural effusion: a prospective, randomized trial*. Med Sci Monit, 2003. 9(6): pp. PI54–59.

[129] Antony, V.B., *Pathogenesis of malignant pleural effusions and talc pleurodesis*. Pneumologie, 1999. 53(10): pp. 493–498.

[130] Alberts, D.S., et al., *Bleomycin pharmacokinetics in man. II. Intracavitary administration*. Cancer Chemother Pharmacol, 1979. 2(2): pp. 127–132.

[131] Yu, H., *Management of pleural effusion, empyema, and lung abscess*. Seminars Intervent Radiol, 2016. 28.1: pp. 75–86.

[132] Rahman, N.M., et al., *Intrapleural use of tissue plasminogen activator and DNase in pleural infection*. N Engl J Med, 2011. 365(6): pp. 518–526.

[133] Piccolo, F., et al., *Intrapleural tissue plasminogen activator and deoxyribonuclease therapy for pleural infection*. J Thorac Dis, 2015. 7(6): pp. 999–1008.

[134] Maskell, N.A., et al., *U.K. controlled trial of intrapleural streptokinase for pleural infection*. N Engl J Med, 2005. 352(9): pp. 865–874.

[135] Liang, C., et al., *Severe intraoperative complications during VATS lobectomy compared with thoracotomy lobectomy for early stage non-small cell lung cancer*. J Thorac Dis, 2013. 5(4): pp. 513–517.

[136] Rostand, R.A., Feldman, R.L. and Block, E.R., *Massive hemothorax complicating heparin anticoagulation for pulmonary embolus*. South Med J, 1977. 70(9): pp. 1128–1130.

[137] Morecroft, J.A. and Lea, R.E., *Haemothorax—a complication of anticoagulation for suspected pulmonary embolism*. Br J Clin Pract, 1988. 42(5): pp. 217–218.

[138] Joseph, J. and Sahn, S.A., *Thoracic endometriosis syndrome: new observations from an analysis of 110 cases*. Am J Med, 1996. 100(2): pp. 164–170.

[139] Elsayed, H., *Haemothorax after mediastinoscopy: a word of caution*. Eur J Cardiothorac Surg, 2012. 41(1): pp. 138139.

[140] McGee, D.C. and Gould, M.K., *Preventing complications of central venous catheterization*. N Engl J Med, 2003. 348(12): pp. 1123–1133.

[141] Patrini, D., et al., *Etiology and management of spontaneous haemothorax*. J Thorac Dis, 2015. 7(3): pp. 520–526.

[142] Wolverson, M.K., et al., *Hyperdensity of recent hemorrhage at body computed tomography: incidence and morphologic variation*. Radiology, 1983. 148(3): pp. 779–784.

[143] Velmahos, G.C., et al., *Predicting the need for thoracoscopic evacuation of residual traumatic hemothorax: chest radiograph is insufficient*. J Trauma, 1999. 46(1): pp. 65–70.

[144] Enderson, B.L., et al., *Tube thoracostomy for occult pneumothorax: a prospective randomized study of its use*. J Trauma, 1993. 35(5): pp. 726–729; discussion 729–730.

[145] Light, R.W., *Pleural Diseases*. 5th ed. Lippincott: Williams and Wilkins, 2007.

[146] Light, R.W. and Lee, Y.C.G., Textbook of Pleural Diseases. 2nd ed. CRC Press, 2008, London, UK, Arnold Hodder.

[147] Light, R.W., et al., *Textbook of Respiratory Diseases: Pneumothorax, Chylothorax, Hemothorax and Fibrothorax*. 5 ed. Philadelphia: Saunders Elsevier, 2010.

[148] Ali, H.A., et al., *Spontaneous hemothorax: a comprehensive review*. Chest, 2008. 134(5): pp. 1056–1065.

[149] Carrillo, E.H. and Richardson, J.D., *Thoracoscopy in the management of hemothorax and retained blood after trauma*. Curr Opin Pulm Med, 1998. 4(4): pp. 243–246.

[150] Landreneau, R.J., et al., *Thoracoscopy for empyema and hemothorax*. Chest, 1996. 109(1): pp. 18–24.

[151] Pollak, J.S. and Passik, C.S., *Intrapleural urokinase in the treatment of loculated pleural effusions*. Chest, 1994. 105(3): pp. 868–873.

[152] Inci, I., et al., *Intrapleural fibrinolytic treatment of traumatic clotted hemothorax*. Chest, 1998. 114(1): pp. 160–165.

[153] Boersma, W.G., Stigt, J.A. and Smit, H.J., *Treatment of haemothorax*. Respir Med, 2010. 104(11): pp. 1583–1587.

[154] Maxwell, R.A., et al., *Use of presumptive antibiotics following tube thoracostomy for traumatic hemopneumothorax in the prevention of empyema and pneumonia--a multi-center trial*. J Trauma, 2004. 57(4): pp. 742–748; discussion 748–749.

Chapter 2

Pharmacologic Considerations in Oncology Critical Care

Trisha Patel, Erica M. McGovern, Denise Wolfe,
Mark E. Lewis and Mashiul Chowdhury

Additional information is available at the end of the chapter

http://dx.doi.org/10.5772/64599

Abstract

Critical care in the oncology population consists of diverse levels of diseases, syndromes, and emergencies that are not observed in typical medically-ill patients and, with it, comes even more specialized treatment strategies. Therefore, the uncommon or less well-understood pharmacologic considerations in this population must be discussed to better assist any clinician at the bedside. This chapter outlines some of the situations commonly encountered in this setting such as the challenge of treating and preventing infectious diseases when the patient lacks the ability to mount appropriate immune responses to conventional therapy, the paradigm of treating thromboembolism in the group of patients who are at highest risk for both bleeding and clotting and treatment of acute and long-term consequences of cancer or chemotherapy requiring escalation of care to the intensive care unit (ICU).

Keywords: pharmacology, pharmacokinetics, pharmacodynamics, treatment, therapy

1. Introduction

Common diseases and syndromes are identified in intensive care unit (ICU) oncology patients secondary to the progression of cancer or chemotherapy. Such challenges include frequent infections, thromboembolism with concomitant bleeding in lieu of sepsis, and toxicity from chemotherapy, leading to emergent ICU admission. The optimal treatment strategies for these syndromes become especially challenging in ICU patients with multi-system organ failure and tenuous clinical status. Furthermore, specific pharmacologic differences exist not only in ICU but more specifically in oncology patients. Therefore, we sought to provide clinicians with information that would help them make the appropriate and safest decisions when selecting therapy for such critically ill patients.

2. Antimicrobial therapy in oncology patients with sepsis

"Patients with cancer have a 30% higher risk for death from sepsis which accounts for approximately 10% of all cancer deaths" [1]. Hematologic cancers (66.4 per 1000) have a higher mortality rate and are more likely to develop severe sepsis compared to solid tumors (7.6 per 1000). The source of sepsis can be related to the site of the primary tumor as observed in the frequency with which lung cancer patients acquire respiratory infections or prostate cancer patients acquire genitourinary infections [1]. Disruption in mucosal and integumentary systems, neutropenia, cellular and humoral immune dysfunction, splenectomy, presences of indwelling vascular catheters, and local tumor effects are some risk factors of developing infection in cancer patients.

It is necessary to understand the preferred regimens so therapy can be tailored to the most likely source of infection. Furthermore, it is crucial to optimize the pharmacodynamics of antimicrobials in critically ill oncology patients to augment outcomes. Outlined here are several of the infectious disease-related phenomena unique to the critically ill oncology population including the treatment regimens. Guidelines should be referenced for the appropriate time to de-escalate or discontinue treatment regimens. Furthermore, primary antibiotic choice should be based on local susceptibility patterns and formulary agents.

2.1. Neurosurgical-related bacterial meningitis

Bacterial meningitis is one of the most common CNS infections in hematopoietic stem cell transplant and neurosurgical patients who are commonly transferred after surgery to the ICU for continued post-op monitoring of intracranial pressure (ICP), cerebral perfusion pressure (CPP), and neurological status. Patients with primary and systemic metastasis from brain tumors who had neurosurgical procedures account for 25% of cancer patients who develop CNS infections. Risk factors include barrier disruption, poor wound healing due to radiation therapy, and those with Ommaya reservoirs frequently used for fluid sampling and chemotherapy. A retrospective study evaluated 146 patients who developed meningitis after undergoing neurosurgery within 1 year. The most common organisms identified to cause the infections were *Staphylococcus epidermidis* (28.1%); *Staphylococcus hominis* (11.0%); *Staphylococcus haemolyticus* (9.6%); *Staphylococcus aureus* (8.2%); and *Enterococcus* (8.2%). *Propionibacter acnes* is another underappreciated gram-positive anaerobe bacteria, which is commonly associated with various types of implant-associated infections including neurosurgical shunts. With *Propionibacter acnes* belonging to the normal skin microbiota, it can easily cause early shunt infections when theses microorganisms are introduced during surgery [2]. Gram-negative bacteria must also be considered in this type of infection with *Klebsiella pneumoniae* (7.5%) being the most common, followed by *Acinetobacter baumannii* (2.1%), *Pseudomonas aeruginosa* (1.4%), and *Escherichia coli* (1.4%). Empiric therapy should consist of a beta-lactam antibiotic that has adequate CNS penetration (i.e., cefepime, meropenem, or ceftazidime) in addition to an agent that covers MRSA (i.e., vancomycin). The agents of choice for the treatment of specific organisms are listed in **Table 1**, along with other common fungi known to cause meningitis in the oncology critically ill patient.

http://dx.doi.org/10.5772/64599

Organism	Primary regimen	Alternative regimen
Ampicillin susceptible Enterococcus species	Ampicillin plus gentamicin	–
Ampicillin resistant Enterococcus species	Vancomycin[1] plus gentamicin	–
Enterococcus species Ampicillin and Vancomycin resistant	Linezolid	–
Escherichia coli and other Enterobacteriaceae	Ceftriaxone or cefotaxime	Aztreonam, Ciprofloxacin, meropenem, SMX/TMP
Listeria monocytogenes	Ampicillin or Pen G	SMX/TMP,, meropenem
Methicillin susceptible Staph aureus	Nafcillin or oxacillin	Vancomycin[1], meropenem
Methicillin resistant Staph aureus	Vancomycin[1]	SMX/TMP, Linezolid
Staphylococcus epidermidis	Vancomycin[1]	Linezolid
Streptococcus pneumoniae	Penicillin MIC <0.1 μg/mL: Pen G or ampicillin 0.1–1 μg/mL: ceftriaxone or cefotaxime ≥2 μg/mL: Vancomycin[1] + ceftriaxone or cefotaxime	Penicillin MIC <0.1 μg/mL: ceftriaxone cefotaxime 0.1–1 μg/mL:, meropenem ≥2 μg/mL: moxifloxacin
Propionibacterium acnes	Vancomycin[1] plus cefepime Vancomycin[1] plus ceftazidime Vancomycin[1] plus meropenem	–
Pseudomonas aeruginosa	Cefepime or ceftazidime	Aztreonam, ciprofloxacin meropenem PLUS Aminoglycoside

Pen, penicillin; SMX/TMP, sulfamethoxazole/trimethoprim.
[1] See vancomycin section for dosing.

Table 1. Agent of choice for bacterial meningitis based on culture identification [3, 4].

2.2. Catheter-associated urinary tract infections

Urinary tract infections (UTIs) are frequently encountered in oncology critically ill patients due to frequent use of indwelling urinary catheters, urological procedures including ureteric stent placements, neutropenia, and prolonged use of steroids. One hospital evaluated 115 patients with advanced cancer who had positive cultures in an eight (8)-month period. As the predominate infection, 61% of UTIs occurred in patients with indwelling catheters. Gram-negative organisms were the most common bacteria isolated, and patients receiving corticosteroids had the highest rate of UTIs [5]. One study included 22 patients with malignancy and found in 57 original ureteric stents, 25 (44%) had bacterial colonization. Not all colonization will lead to true UTIs. However, if the urine culture is positive or the leukocyte count is greater than 30 on urinalysis, then antibiotic use and removal or change of the stent should be considered due to stent colonization [6]. A lack of strong data exists for initiating prolonged prophylactic antibiotics after stent placement to prevent such infections. Therefore, it is important to treat based on whether the patient is symptomatic and an accurate diagnosis of an active infection. Literature on empiric regimens, specifically in the oncology population, is unavailable, and therefore, it is recommended a broad-spectrum beta-lactam antibiotic be used with the addition of an antipseudomonal antibiotic if pseudomonas is suspected. Hemodynamically stable patients may be candidates for single-agent therapy such as a fluoroquinolone. Duration of therapy should be based on clinical response with therapy continued for 10–14 days if response is delayed [7].

2.3. Post-obstructive pneumonia

Post-obstructive pneumonia is frequently encountered in patients with cancer and can quickly lead to ICU admission if symptoms become severe. This type of pneumonia is defined as a "radiographic opacification resulting from complete or partial airway obstruction by a pulmonary neoplasm" [8]. The findings can be a result of non-infectious (mucus plugging, parenchymal inflammation, or tumor) or infectious causes. Patients will often present with severe cough, wheezing, and dyspnea, but these symptoms can be misleading making it difficult to determine the need for antibiotic therapy. For example, patients may not have signs of infection such as fever, chills, and leukocytosis and still have a microbe isolated. More commonly, an infection is present if the patient has an infiltrate in addition to a fever [8]. The majority of post-obstructive pneumonias are polymicrobial caused by *Haemophilus influenza, Klebsiella pneumonia, Enterobacter cloacae, Acinetobacter* species, *Pseudomonas aeruginosa, Staphylococcus aureus*, and *Streptococcus viridans*. Management of such infections requires treating the source of obstruction through interventional bronchoscopy techniques in addition to antimicrobial therapy. Until cultures are identified, a broad-spectrum gram-negative agent (i.e., cefepime) in addition to MRSA coverage should be initiated based on local susceptibility patterns. Treatment should be considered for at least 7–10 days, similar to health-care-associated pneumonias and based on patient's clinical improvement.

2.4. Fever in the oncology patient

In both the critically ill and cancer patient, fever can be a common symptom not always secondary to infection. Among 371 patients (477 episodes), fever was identified due to non-infectious causes in 23% of patients and due to unknown origin in 10% of patients [9]. Non-infectious causes, independent of tumors, can be related to an allergic reaction, thromboembolism, or an inflammatory disease. Cancer-related fever is classically associated with non-Hodgkin's and Hodgkin's lymphoma, leukemia, and solid tumors [10]. A recent study defined tumor fever as no microbiological, radiological, or clinical evidence of infection and lack of response to empirical antimicrobial therapy for at least 7 days or experienced a positive response to a naproxen test. Using this definition, the investigators evaluated the role of a procalcitonin (PCT) test for differentiating infectious from non-infectious fever in non-neutropenic patients. The baseline PCT level was not different between those with tumor-related fever and blood stream infections. However, there was a statistically significant difference in the decrease in PCT levels between the two groups in response to antimicrobials suggesting one method for differentiating fever due to infectious versus non-infectious causes [11]. Other sources of fever which must be considered are chemotherapy (azathioprine, hydroxyurea, interleukin-2, rituximab, and interferon), transfusions, surgery, or procedures [9, 10]. Drug-induced fever is often overlooked and should be highly considered especially if the fever resolves after stopping the expected culprit. Such medications in the ICU that should be evaluated in the patient are antimicrobials, succinylcholine or inhaled anesthetics antipsychotics possibly causing neuroleptic malignant syndrome, or antidepressants leading to serotonin syndrome [12]. Fever in these patients may not present in any particular pattern, and signs of infection are attenuated due to the decreased inflammatory response so fever tends to be the only sign of ensuing infection. Therefore, it is imperative to identify fever associated with other symptoms such as rigors and chills to suggest an infectious source and initiate appropriate targeted therapy.

2.5. Vancomycin dosing in oncology patients

Since the 1950s, studies have evaluated the pharmacokinetic (PK) and pharmacodynamic (PD) profile of vancomycin to determine the best parameter that predicts its efficacy in clinical practice. National guidelines provide broad recommendations, which should be applied as the foundation for creating institution level policies [13]. However, they lack recommendations specific to oncology patients, whose vancomycin PK is greatly altered when compared to the general population. Furthermore, critically ill patients are subject to frequent alterations in drug PK due to fluctuations in creatinine clearance, shifting of fluid leading to changes in volume of distribution, decreased tissue perfusion, and decreased metabolism with organ dysfunction all of which must be accounted for when dosing antibiotics. Several pharmacokinetic (PK) studies have shown an increased vancomycin volume of distribution (Vd) and clearance (Cl) in cancer patients, requiring these patients to receive nearly double the average dose than patients without cancer (60 vs. 30 mg/kg/day) to obtain therapeutic levels [14]. More specific data with regards to cancer type or other patient factors contributing to these changes have not been elucidated.

The PD parameter that best reflects clinical efficacy of vancomycin against *S. aureus is* AUC/MIC with a target of ≥400 h [13, 15]. It has been proposed that 3–4 g of vancomycin per day would be required for 90% probability of attaining an AUC/MIC of 400 h for an MIC of 1 mg/L and ≥5 g per day for vancomycin-intermediate susceptible *S. aureus* (VISA) strains [13]. However, readily calculating the AUC/MIC is challenging and cannot easily be performed. Subsequently, most clinical pharmacists have continued to use trough levels for determining therapeutic concentrations. Therefore, until more efficient tools are available for applying pharmacodynamics methods with AUC/MIC, it is suggested that multiple daily doses (three or four as opposed to two with same total daily dose) may be preferred to achieve target therapeutic levels in patients with hematologic malignancy and normal renal function [16]. In the critically ill patient, vancomycin can be also be effected by augmented renal clearance (ARC) due to sepsis, trauma, autoimmune disorders, or major surgery. With AUC inversely related to renal clearance, ARC can extensively impact the PK of vancomycin and lead to subtherapeutic levels [17]. These combined factors in both oncology and critically ill patients further support the need for possibly higher doses in this population.

2.6. Extended-infusion beta-lactam therapy

Studies have shown improvement in clinical outcomes (i.e., patient survival and duration of hospitalization after onset of infection) by optimizing the pharmacodynamics with use of extended-infusion (EI) dosing regimens. The best predictor of bacterial killing for β-lactams is the time during which the free drug concentration exceeds the MIC of the organism ($fT > MIC$). Near-maximal β-lactams bactericidal effect is typically observed when the free drug concentration exceeds the MIC for 50%, and 40% of the dosing interval for penicillins and carbapenems, respectively [18–20]. With the increase in resistance among gram-negative organisms, optimizing activity of β-lactam antibiotics through dosing strategies becomes crucial to preserve clinical efficacy.

Of the most common β-lactams used in critically ill oncology patients, piperacillin–tazobactam and meropenem administered via extended infusion are associated with the most positive clinical outcomes and have a higher probability of achieving target attainment. One retrospective study assessed 194 patients who received 3.375 g IV every 4 or 6 h over a 30-min infusion, vs. 3.375 g IV every 8 h over a 4-h infusion for treatment of *P. aeruginosa* infections. Higher mortality and longer length of stay were seen with intermittent infusions (31.6% of patients) compared to EI (12.2% of patients) in the more critically ill patients. Furthermore, the Monte Carlo simulation showed the probability of target attainment (PTA) was only 20% with intermittent infusion vs. 100% PTA with EI at an MIC of 16. With the MIC breakpoint for *P. aeruginosa* to PTZ being ≤16/4, it is evident that intermittent infusions may not achieve optimal levels to be efficacious [18].

Creatinine clearance (mL/min)	Dose
Extended infusion	
≥20 mL/min	3.375 g (30-min infusion) × 1 dose STAT Followed by 3.375 gm IV q8 h via 4 h infusion
<20 mL/min (including IHD/PD)	3.375 g (30-min infusion) × 1 dose STAT, 3.375 g IV q12 h via 4 h infusion
CRRT	3.375 g (30-min infusion) × 1 dose STAT, 3.375 gm IV q8 h via 4 h infusion

CRRT, continuous renal replacement therapy; PD, peritoneal dialysis; IHD, intermittent hemodialysis.

Table 2. Extended and conventional Piperacillin-tazobactam dosing [22].

The use of loading doses prior to initiating extended infusion and time to exceeding the MIC breakpoint has also been studied. A PK model demonstrated that 90% of the patients would be expected to have PTZ and meropenem drug concentrations exceed the MIC breakpoint within 6 min if both agents were preceded by a loading dose versus 8 h and 36 min, respectively, without a loading dose [21]. Therefore, with sepsis guidelines providing evidence to support a mortality benefit in administering antibiotics within 60 min for patients in septic shock, a loading dose should be highly considered. Loading doses may be less important for meropenem and susceptible organisms as optimal drug concentrations were achieved with any regimen in no later than 36 min [21]. From the evidence outlined, the dosing regimens for PTZ listed in **Table 2** are recommended for critically ill oncology patients.

A retrospective, pre/post-observation study of intermittent vs. extended-infusion meropenem was conducted in hematopoietic stem-cell transplant patients and those treated with induction chemotherapy for AML. Meropenem 1 g every 8 h via short 30-min infusion (SI) was compared with 1 g every 8 h via extended 4-h infusion (EI). After 5 days of treatment, therapy was successful in more cases in the EI group than the SI group (69.4 vs. 40.9%, $p = 0.001$) [23]. Various meropenem regimens were also reviewed in a Monte Caro simulation. The probability of achieving drug concentrations above the MIC for >40% of the dosing interval for *Pseudomonas aeruginosa* were 87.9, 93.5, and 96.7% for doses of 500, 1000, and 2000 mg, respectively, and thus, higher doses may be needed for immunocompromised patients with bacteria exhibiting higher meropenem MICs (e.g., MIC >4 mg/L) [24]. Minimal evidence is available on the appropriate dosage adjustments in renal failure. However, one study did evaluate the effects of augmented renal clearance in critically ill patients on achieving target attainments with extended-infusion meropenem (1 g IV every 8 h via 3-h infusion). Patients with a creatinine clearance (CrCl) of 50 mL/min had a predicted probability of target attainment of approximately 90% which inversely declined with increases in creatinine clearance (fT > MIC of ~50 and ~20% at CrCl of 100 and 150 mL/min, respectively). Therefore, critically ill patients who commonly exhibit augmented clearance should have dosing regimens optimized whenever feasible with lower doses possibly not considered until the CrCl is less than or equal to 50 mL/min [25]. Consequently, we would recommend a regimen of meropenem 2 g IV every 8 h via 3-h infusion for most critically ill oncology patients.

2.7. Treatment of multi-drug resistant organisms

As stated by the CDC, "antimicrobial resistance is one of our most serious health threats" [26]. The rate of infections caused by gram-negative organisms continues to rise and significantly contribute to morbidity and mortality worldwide [27]. First- and second-line antibiotics are no longer effective for such organisms, and thus, efforts to discover and approve new antimicrobials continue to strengthen. The patient populations deemed to be most vulnerable to resistant organisms are those receiving chemotherapy, recent hospital and intensive care unit admission, and those with invasive devices. Due to their frequent exposure to antibiotics and hospitalizations, risk of acquiring such organisms is significantly increased. Much of the data for treatment of multi-drug resistant organisms are based on case studies or retrospective studies. The multitude of data concerning appropriate treatment options for all multi-drug resistant organisms exceeds the capacity of this chapter. Therefore, primary and secondary regimens for only CRE and ESBL organisms have been described in **Tables 3** and **4**.

Infection	Regimen options
UTI	Ceftazidime/avibactam 2.5 g IV q8 h
	Fosfomycin One packet (3 grams) orally q2 to 3 days for 3 doses (can be extended to 21 days in some cases)
	Meropenem IV 2 g q8 h (3-h infusion)[3] plus Ertapenem 1 g IV q24 h (1 h after meropenem)
	Colistin IV[1,2,4] plus Meropenem 2 g q8 h (3-h infusion)[3]
Bacteremia	Colistin IV[2,4] plus Meropenem IV 2 g q8 h (3-h infusion)[3]
	Polymixin B[2] plus Meropenem 2 g IV q8 h (3-h infusion)[3]
Intra-abdominal	Ceftazidime/avibactam 2.5 g IV q8 h plus Metronidazole 500 mg IV q8 h
	Colistin IV[2,4] plus Meropenem 2 g q8 h (3 h infusion)[3]
	Polymixin B[2] plus Meropenem 2 g IV q8 h (3 h infusion)[3] plus Tigecycline 200 mg IV loading dose then 100 mg IV q12 to 24 h if meropenem MIC >16 mcg/mL and polymyxin B MIC >2 mcg/mL
ASSSI	Tigecycline 200 mg IV loading dose then 100 mg IV q12 to 24 h plus Polymixin B[2] plus Meropenem 2 g q8 h (3-h infusion)[3]

ASSSI, acute skin/skin structure infection; UTI, urinary tract infection.
[1] Colistin IV is recommended over Polymixin B for treatment of urinary tract infections based on pharmacokinetic properties. Urinary concentrations of Polymixin B remain low compared to Colistin due to Polymixin B is eliminated primarily by non-renal mechanisms.
[2] Refer to references [33] and [96] for appropriate dosing.
[3] Monitor patient closely for development of seizures with high-dose carbapenems.
[4] Not recommended for organism with MIC ≥4.

Table 3. Regimens for treatment of CRE by site of infection [25, 28–33].

Antimicrobial	Comments
Carbapenem (imipenem, meropenem, ertapenem)	First-line agents
Ceftolozane/tazobactam Ceftazidime/avibactam (add Metronidazole for intra-abdominal infections)	Only indicated for treatment of complicated intra-abdominal infections and complicated urinary tract infections including pyelonephritis (*in vitro data*)
Tigecycline	Only indicated for treatment of complicated skin and skin structure infections, complicated intra-abdominal infections, and community-acquired pneumonia Limited penetration in urinary tract and blood
β-lactam/β-lactamase inhibitor combinations (amoxicillin-clavulanate, piperacillin–tazobactam, ampicillin-sulbactam)	Such agents should be reserved for treatment of ESBL organisms from the urinary tract with poor efficacy data for other sites of infections due to these organisms
Colistin	High-risk for renal toxicity
Fosfomycin	IV formulation not available in the USA Oral formulation only indicated for UTI

Table 4. Antimicrobial therapy regimens for treatment of extended-spectrum beta-lactamases (ESBL) [34–36].

http://dx.doi.org/10.5772/64599

2.8. Clostridium difficile infection (CDI)

The rates of CDI continue to increase exponentially with strains becoming more virulent and difficult to treat in addition to more patients becoming colonized. Oncology patients, especially those with hematological malignancies, are particularly susceptible due to multiple risk factors such as frequent and prolonged hospitalizations, exposure to multiple courses of antibiotics, and chemotherapeutic agents. It has even been proposed that chemotherapeutic agents without concomitant antibiotics have been associated with CDI. Such incidences are most commonly reported to be caused by methotrexate and 5-FU. Methotrexate is suspected to cause severe disruption of intestinal protein metabolism causing a pronounced inflammatory cytokine response and promoting CDI. Similar effects have been seen due to irinotecan and topotecan; thus, clinicians should monitor for signs of CDI even after chemotherapy administration. Appropriate diagnostic work-ups with combination testing (i.e., glutamate dehydrogenase followed by confirmatory testing with enzyme immunoassay and quantitative real-time PCR) should be performed to differentiate between colonization and true infections (**Figures 1** and **2**) [95].

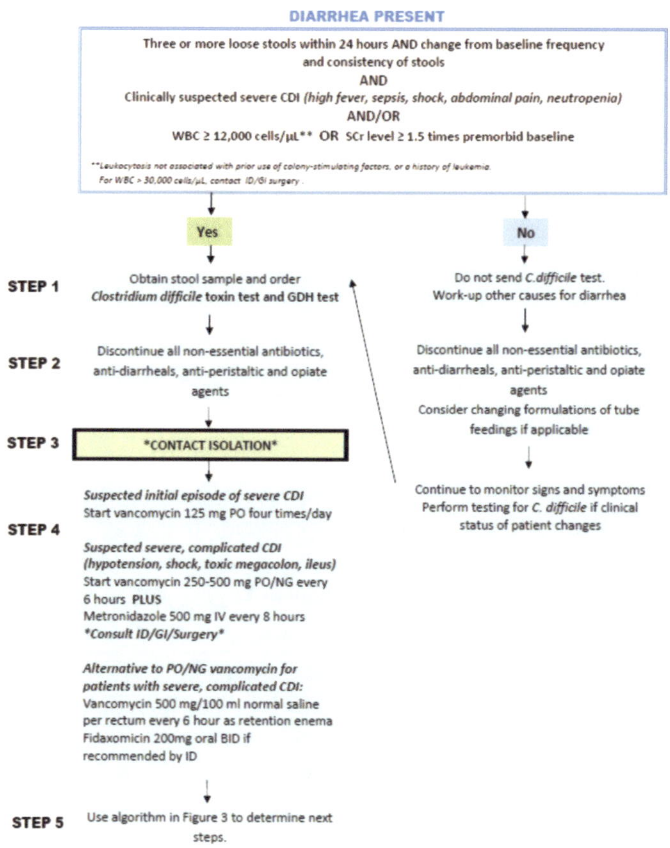

Figure 1. Diagnosis and Treatment of CDI.

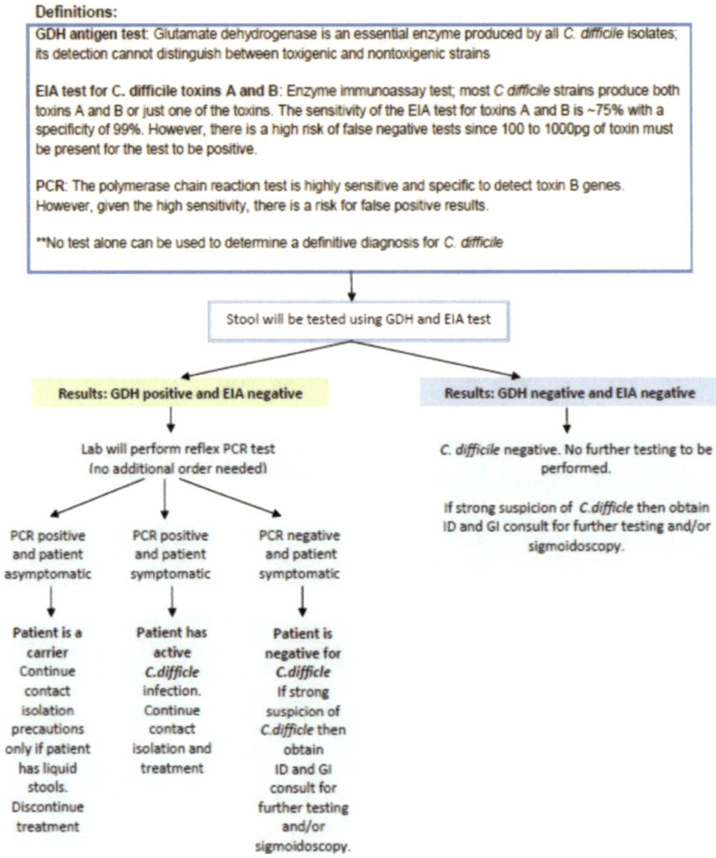

Figure 2. Appropriate *C.difficile* Testing and Interpretation.

2.9. Intra-abdominal infections

Intra-abdominal infections in cancer patients are especially common following surgery. One of the high-risk procedures being performed in several oncology centers is hyperthermic intraperitoneal chemotherapy (HIPEC) which can be associated with severe complications such as peritonitis. These patients are often transferred to the ICU for post-op monitoring and thus the ICU becomes the unit where such infections are managed. A retrospective study noted 9% of 52 patients required reoperation for post-operative peritonitis following complete cytoreductive surgery (CCRS) combined with HIPEC. The infections were most frequently caused by *E. coli* in 5 samples (71%) and Enterobacter species in two samples (29%), with seven of the nine bacteriological species being multi-drug resistant. Unfortunately, this is only one of the many intra-abdominal infections these patients can experience.

In the elderly population (>65 years), it was noted that the spectra of diseases that cause intra-abdominal sepsis are different from younger populations. The most common types in the elderly were diverticulitis, cholecystitis, cholangitis, and perforation of the colon from obstructing adenocarcinoma. Advanced tumors leading to perforation and then abscesses or peritonitis have been reported as frequently as 2.6–10%. This can quickly lead to severe sepsis or septic shock that requires management in the ICU. The common offending organisms identified are those of the gastrointestinal tract, *Enterococcus* species, *Candida* species, *Staphylococcus epidermidis, E. coli, Enterobacter* species, *B. fragilis*, and *Pseudomonas* species [40]. There are no guidelines available for recommendations on antimicrobial therapy specific to critically ill oncology patients, and therefore, it is recommended that combination therapy is initiated with a broad-spectrum agent with anaerobic coverage, a second gram-negative agent with activity against *Pseudomonas aeruginosa* if suspected, and an antifungal agent with activity against *Candida glabrata*.

Per IDSA guidelines, it is recommended that intravenous (IV) metronidazole is added to vanco-26mycin oral only in the "severe, complicated" cases defined by hypotension, shock, the presence of an ileus, or megaco-27lon, and not in "severe" cases (white blood cell (WBC) count of ≥15,000 cells/mL or serum creatinine ≥1.5 times base-28line) [37]. A recent retrospective, observational study evaluated mortality amongst critically ill patients who received 29 oral vancomycin vs. oral vancomycin with IV metronidazole defined by primarily clinical criteria. A total of 88 pa?30tients were evaluated including 23 immunocompromised patients. Mortality were found to be significantly better in31the combination therapy group, compared to the monotherapy group (36.4 vs. 15.9%, p = 0.03). This suggests the need32to further consider the true definition of "severe disease" vs. "critically ill" and whether selection of therapy should be33based on clinical criteria in addition to laboratory data. The study design cannot definitively provide support for all34critically ill patients receiving combination therapy; however, it does propose that IV metronidazole in addition to van-35comycin should be considered in the most severely ill patients [38]. Per IDSA guidelines, it is recommended that intravenous (IV) metronidazole is added to vanco-26mycin oral only in the "severe, complicated" cases defined by hypotension, shock, the presence of an ileus, or megaco-27lon, and not in "severe" cases (white blood cell (WBC) count of ≥15,000 cells/mL or serum creatinine ≥1.5 times base-28line) [37].

The administration of probiotics is also a common topic amongst patients who are on prolonged antibiotic2therapy for primary or secondary prevention of C. difficile. As IDSA guidelines recommended in 2010, there are limited3data to support its use and potential risk for bloodstream infections [37]. A report released by the World Health Organ-4ization (WHO) noted probiotics may be theoretically responsible for four types of side effects: (1) systemic infections,5(2) deleterious metabolic activities, (3) excessive immune stimulation in susceptible individuals, and (4) gene transfer.6There have been several case reports of infections caused by organisms consistent with probiotic strains including but7not limited to Saccharomyces boulardii, Lactobacilli, Lactobacillus acidophilus, and Lactobacillus casei [39]. Due to the use of8probiotics remaining controversial and with the lack of clinical trials to confirm the safety of these products, clinicians9are advised to remain cautious when using such products in immunocompromised patients, including those started on 10 corticosteroids, which is common in ICU patients [39].

Empiric regimens for necrotizing fasciitis	
Primary regimen	Alternative regimen
Piperacillin–tazobactam extended infusion (preferred) or intermittent infusion plus vancomycin[1]	Levofloxacin plus (clindamycin or metronidazole) plus aminoglycoside
Imipenem-cilastatin	
Meropenem	
Ertapenem	
Cefotaxime plus metronidazole or clindamycin	
Regimens based on culture data	
Streptococcus	Penicillin plus clindamycin
Clostridium species	
Aeromonas hydrophila	Doxycycline plus (ciprofloxacin or ceftriaxone)
Vibrio vulnificus	Doxycycline plus (ceftriaxone or cefotaxime)
Gram-negative organisms	Based on local susceptibility (Carbapenem for ESBL-producing organisms)

[1] See vancomycin section for dosing.

Table 5. Treatment regimens for necrotizing fasciitis [44].

2.10. Skin and soft tissue infections

Chemotherapy, radiation, and multiple surgical procedures place oncology patients at risk for developing skin and soft tissue infections. One particularly lethal skin infection that requires immediate transfer to the ICU is necrotizing fasciitis (NF) which has been more commonly associated with certain debilitating conditions such as immunosuppression. No true risk factors have been delineated, and the cause of ≥20% of necrotizing soft tissue infections is idiopathic making it challenging to determine precipitating factors. The onset and progression of signs and symptoms are rapid especially with Group A *Streptococcus* or *Clostridium* making it crucial that both surgical intervention and antibiotic intervention are considered immediately when suspecting NF [41]. In a retrospective review with 8534 hematological malignancy patients, nine (9) were diagnosed with NF. Interestingly, pathogens isolated were all gram-negative organisms (*Salmonella, Vibrio vulnificus, Aeromonas*, ESBL *Klebsiella*, ESBL *Escherichia coli*, and *Enterobacter cloacae*) [42]. Another case report was published of a febrile neutropenia patient with myelodysplastic syndrome (MDS) that experienced a blunt injury to the left upper extremity. This resulted in rapid progression of the wound with fluid accumulation that extended from the left upper arm to the proximal medial forearm. All blood cultures revealed *S. maltophilia*, and the patient was treated both surgically and with IV trimethoprim/sulfamethoxazole [43]. Although group A *Streptococcus* has

http://dx.doi.org/10.5772/64599

most commonly been known as the leading cause of NF, more than one retrospective review has identified gram-negative NF associated with malignancy making it imperative for clinicians to consider broad-spectrum antibiotics that adequately cover for possible resistant organisms as shown in **Table 5** [42].

Another common skin infection in oncology patients known to be closely related to lymphedema is cellulitis. Unfortunately, every incidence of cellulitis can further damage the lymphatic system which in turn leads to secondary episodes of lymphedema. Due to the protein-rich lymphatic fluid which accumulates due to impaired drainage, bacteria can easily invade such areas and cause local cellulitis infections. Therapy should be directed at likely organisms such as *streptococcus* and patients with three to four episodes per year of recurrent cellulitis should be considered for prophylactic antibiotics (~4–52 weeks) [44, 45]. As suggested by IDSA guidelines, non-purulent soft tissue skin infections in immunocompromised patients are categorized as "severe" and should be considered for broader therapy with piperacillin–tazobactam plus vancomycin [44]. Purulent skin and soft tissue infections should undergo incision and drainage with the addition of antibiotics (**Figure 3**).

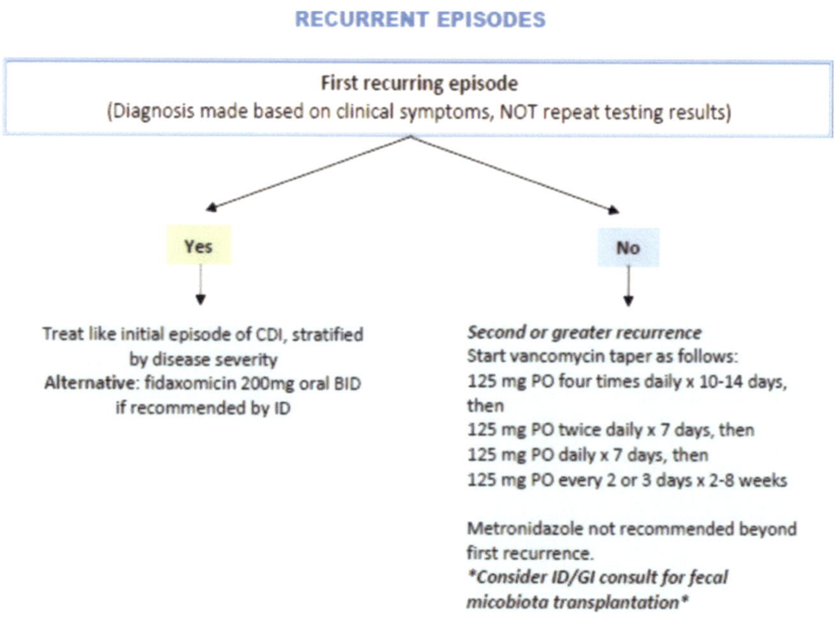

Figure 3. Treatment Algorithm of Recurrent Episodes.

The ideal treatment options for the numerous infections that oncology critical care patients encounter have yet to be defined. Subsequently, therapy should always be optimized with respect to pharmacokinetic and pharmacodynamic properties of antimicrobials when regimens are selected. It is also well understood that therapy is often most aggressive in the immunocompromised and severely ill population. Therefore, side effects and toxicities of all agents must be weighed against efficacy to ensure safety is not compromised.

3. Prophylactic and therapeutic anticoagulation

3.1. Epidemiology

It is well known that the risk of thrombosis in oncology patients far exceeds the risk encountered by those without a cancer diagnosis. Thrombosis accounts for 10% of fatal events in oncology patients, making it the second leading cause of death in this patient population. Patients with cancer experience between a twofold to 20-fold increased risk of developing venous thromboembolism (VTE), which is most likely to occur within the first six months of cancer diagnosis [46, 47]. Patients diagnosed with cancer of the pancreas, stomach, colon, brain, lung, and ovaries are at higher risk of developing VTE in addition to treatment with antiangiogenic agents, such as thalidomide and lenalidomide used in multiple myeloma [46–49]. Unfortunately, this VTE risk is only further exacerbated in critically ill ICU patients. It has been noted that the incidence of deep venous thrombosis ranges from 28 to 32% in general medical ICU patients with nearly 95% being clinically silent [50]. One single-center prospective cohort identified four risk factors for ICU-acquired VTE including personal or family history of VTE, end-stage renal failure, platelet transfusion, and vasopressor use [51]. Catheters may be subject to thrombotic events, leading to pulmonary embolism in 10–15% of patients and loss of access in 10% of patients [52]. Such complications place a patient in danger of the effects of VTE and impede cancer-directed therapy, enabling progression of the disease.

Not only do VTEs affect a patient's cancer prognosis, but they also increase the risk of complications, such as bleeding, which is 2.5 times more likely to occur in oncology patients receiving anticoagulant therapy within the first year of VTE [46, 48]. Unfortunately, this does not preclude patients from being at risk for recurrence of thrombosis during anticoagulant therapy. Thrombosis during anticoagulant therapy occurs in 6–17% of cancer-related VTE, nearly three times higher than in non-oncology patients with a history of thromboembolism [46–48]. Given the increased risk of VTE in oncology patients contributing to morbidity and prolonged hospitalizations, it is important to adequately understand the options available for treatment and the recommended guidelines for the use of such medications in an oncology population.

3.2. Thromboprophylaxis and first-line treatment

Several well-published guidelines provide recommendations for prophylaxis and treatment of thrombosis in oncology and ICU patients, all of which have slightly different suggestions for appropriate therapy. Thus, it was necessary to provide summaries for several of these publications to allow clinicians to consider multiple view points and make the best clinical decision. Recommendations only applicable to the critically ill oncology population are provided for thromboprophylaxis, treatment of established VTE, and recurrence management in **Tables 6–8**. Additionally, per CHEST guidelines, mechanical prophylaxis alone should be considered only in ICU patients at high risk of bleeding with pharmacologic agents resumed when such bleeding risks are resolved [55]. Combination of pharmacologic and mechanical modalities should be considered in all patients as a meta-analysis published in the Cochrane Library suggested the combination was superior to either alone [58].

Criteria	Prophylaxis options
Non-surgical	
General ICU or hospitalized patients with active malignancy and acute medical illness or reduced mobility. (Not routinely recommended for patients admitted for minor procedures, short chemotherapy infusion, or patients undergoing stem-cell/bone marrow transplantation)	Unfractionated heparin 5000 units SQ q8 h Dalteparin 5000 SQ units daily Enoxaparin 40 mg SQ daily Fondaparinux 2.5 mg SQ daily
Surgery	
All patients with malignant disease undergoing major surgical intervention unless contraindicated because of active bleeding or high bleeding risk.	Unfractionated heparin 5000 units 2–4 h preoperatively and once q8 h thereafter or 5000 units 10–12 h preoperatively and 5000 units twice daily thereafter
Prophylaxis should be continued for at least 7–10 days in patients undergoing major surgery, and up to 4 weeks in patients receiving major abdominal and pelvic surgery with high-risk factors such as restricted mobility, obesity, history of VTE, or with additional risk factors noted in ASCO guidelines.[1]	Dalteparin 2500 units SQ 2–4 h preoperatively and 5000 units SQ daily thereafter or 5,000 units SQ 10–12 h preoperatively and 5000 units SQ once daily thereafter Enoxaparin 20 mg SQ 2–4 h preoperatively and 40 g daily thereafter or 40 mg SQ 10–12 h preoperatively and 40 mg SQ once daily thereafter
LMWH or UFH commenced	Fondaparinux 2.5 mg SQ daily beginning 6–8 h post-operatively
Post-operatively for the prevention of VTE in oncology patients undergoing neurosurgery.	Additional recommendations for when to initiate prophylactic therapy post-surgery is available through NCCN guidelines

UFH, unfractionated heparin; LMWH, low molecular weight heparin; VTE, venous thromboembolism; SQ, subcutaneous.

[1] Multiple risk assessment models have been proposed but yet to be validated before strong recommendations are made for inpatient screening. ASCO guidelines should be referenced for predictive models.

Table 6. Thromboprophylaxis [52–56].

Criteria	Treatment options
LMWH is preferred over UFH for the initial 5–10 days of anticoagulation for VTE in patients without renal impairment (CrCl <30 mL/min)	Unfractionated heparin 80 units/kg IV bolus, then 18 U/kg per h IV; adjust dose based on aPTT
	Dalteparin 100 units/kg SQ q12 h or 200 units/kg SQ daily
	Enoxaparin 1 mg/kg SQ q12 h or 1.5 mg/kg daily
	Fondaparinux <50 kg: 5 mg SQ daily
	50–100 kg: 7.5 mg SQ daily
	>100 kg: 10 mg SQ daily

Criteria	Treatment options
For long-term anticoagulation (at least 6 months), LMWH is preferred over VKAs (VKA is acceptable if LMWH is not available)	Dalteparin 200 units/kg SQ daily for 1 month, then 150 units/kg SQ daily
Consider anticoagulation beyond 6 months for patients with active cancer (metastatic disease) or those receiving chemotherapy	Enoxaparin 1.5 mg/kg SQ daily or 1 mg/kg once q12 h
For catheter-associated thrombosis, anticoagulate as long as the catheter is in place for at least 3 months	Warfarin Adjust dose to maintain INR 2–3
Consider insertion of vena cava filter in patients with contraindications to anticoagulant therapy or as adjunct to anticoagulation in patients with progression of thrombosis.	
Use of novel oral anticoagulants for either prevention or treatment of VTE in patients with cancer is not formally recommended by national guidelines at this time.	

CrCl, creatinine clearance; UFH, unfractionated heparin; LMWH, low molecular weight heparin; VKA, vitamin K antagonist; VTE, venous thromboembolism.

Table 7. Treatment of newly established VTE [52–54, 57].

Treatment patient was receiving when recurrence of VTE diagnosed	Secondary treatment options
VKA	LMWH[6] or fondaparinux or UFH
LMWH	Increase the dose of LMWH dose in patients treated with LMWH Consider twice daily dosing if patient experiences recurrent VTE while receiving once-daily dosing of LMWH
UFH	LMWH or fondaparinux Increase dose of UFH
Failure of any agent	Consider placement of an inferior vena cava filter

UFH, unfractionated heparin; LMWH, low molecular weight heparin; VKA, vitamin K antagonist; VTE, venous thromboembolism.

Table 8. Treatment of VTE recurrence in oncology patients receiving anticoagulation [52, 54].

3.3. Direct oral anticoagulants (DOACs)

Alternatives to treatment include new, direct oral anticoagulants (DOACs) dabigatran, rivaroxaban, apixaban, and edoxaban. Limited research has been conducted on their use in patients with cancer and the critically ill population [47]. While the standard approach to treating VTE is currently with use of LMWH or fondaparinux followed by warfarin, DOACs simplify anticoagulation therapy as they are administered in fixed doses and do not require routine monitoring [59, 60]. Warfarin therapy, though effective, is accompanied by burdensome disadvantages, including constant monitoring due to the small therapeutic window and multiple drug interactions [60]. Large clinical trials have proven the DOACs to be non-inferior to LMWH/warfarin therapies in efficacy, are associated with fewer bleeding events, and have fewer food/drug interactions [60, 61]. Although the Food and Drug Administration (FDA) has approved rivaroxaban, apixaban, dabigatran, and edoxaban in the USA, the use of DOACs is not formally recommended in oncology patients due to limited clinical data [61]. Furthermore, the use of DOACs especially in ICU should be considered only for those patients who are clinically stable and are not scheduled to have a procedure in the ICU. Despite the lack of randomized trials, many clinicians are beginning to incorporate such oral agents into long-term treatment options for oncology patients due to their ease of administration compared to warfarin and LMWH.

Rivaroxaban is a direct factor Xa inhibitor and was the first DOAC approved by the FDA in 2012 [61–63]. It is contraindicated with inhibitors of CYP3A4 and P-glycoprotein including ketoconazole and ritonavir due to increased plasma drug concentrations [62]. Two non-inferiority studies that included patients with cancer, proved rivaroxaban equally as effective as LMWH/warfarin therapy with similar rates of bleeding [61, 63]. Recurrent VTE occurred in 3.4% of oncology patients treated with rivaroxaban compared to 5.6% of oncology patients with enoxaparin/VKA therapy [63]. One concern with rivaroxaban in critically ill oncology patients is that doses of 15–20 mg must be taken with food to optimize bioavailability. This is often difficult in an oncology population known to have poor appetites and inadequate oral intake. The tablets can be crushed and administered via nasogastric feeding tubes; however, administration via this route must be followed by enteral feedings to optimize absorption. Furthermore, administration through feed tubes placed distal to the stomach will decrease absorption of rivaroxaban [63].

Apixaban, a direct factor Xa inhibitor, was approved by the FDA in 2014 [61]. Similar to rivaroxaban, apixaban is contraindicated with CYP3A4 inhibitors due to increased plasma drug concentrations [62]. In the double-dummy, double-blind AMPLIFY trial, apixaban was proven non-inferior compared to standard anticoagulation therapy (LMWH/warfarin) for incidence of recurrent VTE, and major bleeding events occurred less frequently with apixaban [61]. In the AMPLIFY-EXT trial, long-term anticoagulation for approximately 1 year with apixaban was evaluated in patients who had already been treated for DVT and/or PE for six to 12 months. Compared to placebo, apixaban was superior in preventing recurrent VTE and all-cause death. One additional compelling study evaluating patients with non-valvular atrial fibrillation was able to prove that apixiban 5 mg twice daily compared to aspirin 81–324 mg daily showed significant reduction in stroke and systemic embolism in addition to lower rates of bleeding. The AMPLIFY and AMPLIFY-EXT included a small portion of oncology patients (3.1 and 1.7%, respectively) in which recurrent VTE and major bleeding events occurred about half as frequently in the apixaban group compared to oncology patients treated with enoxaparin/warfarin [64]. Apixaban is further advantageous in ICU patients at risk of multi-system organ failure as it does not require renal or hepatic dosage adjustments.

Dabigatran, a direct thrombin inhibitor, was approved by the FDA in 2014 [61]. Dabigatran proved non-inferior in efficacy and had similar bleeding risks compared to warfarin in the double-blind, double-dummy RE-COVER and RE-COVER II studies [61]. When compared to enoxaparin, rivaroxaban, and apixaban, efficacy was similar but bleeding risks were significantly higher with dabigatran. A meta-analysis comparing trials of these DOACs found that major bleeding risk was lower in those using apixaban than users of dabigatran and edoxaban [65]. Aside from the higher bleeding risk, clinicians should be cautious with its use in the oncology setting as it has a long half-life and requires discontinuation of therapy at least 1–2 days prior to surgery or even as early as 3–5 days for those with a CrCl <50 mL/min. The oral anticoagulant is not recommended for most indications in patients with a CrCl <30 mL/min and must be adjusted if administered with specific P-gp inhibitors. Due to multiple safety risks, the use of dabigatran in the oncology setting has fallen out of favor and caution is advised when treating patients who arrive to the ICU on chronic dabigatran therapy.

Few national guidelines have incorporated these agents into recommendations for treating VTE; however, a recent meta-analysis of five randomized controlled trials did prove that DOACs are comparable to VKA (warfarin) therapy in treating cancer-related VTE, which makes this class of anticoagulants promising in the future [61]. Unfortunately, the DOACs still face one major concern: managing real-world DOAC-associated bleeding, as no antidote is currently FDA-approved for these agents. Some guidelines make recommendations for managing DOAC-associated bleeding events, but the principles are based on laboratory, not clinical parameters [60]. Further research is needed to validate the use of DOACs in VTE treatment, especially in an oncology population.

3.4. Bleeding and thrombocytopenia

Thromboprophylaxis significantly reduces the rate of symptomatic VTE and is important for improving the quality of life in oncology patients, but it is associated with an increased risk of bleeding especially in ICU patients with coagulopathies abnormalities from sepsis and organ failure [48]. In patients with a high risk of bleeding who experience acute proximal DVT or PE, anticoagulation therapy may not be appropriate. The American College of Chest Physicians (ACCP) advises placing an IVC filter in this situation [61].

One common risk for bleeding in oncology critically ill patients is thrombocytopenia secondary to chemotherapy, blood loss during surgery, toxins including other drugs, macrophage-activation syndrome, disseminated intravascular coagulopathy, and massive transfusions. Anticoagulation therapy should be pursued if the platelet count remains above 50×10^9, and platelet transfusions should be considered during the high-risk period of recurrence in order to provide full anticoagulation therapy. Furthermore, it is crucial to delineate whether the cause of thrombocytopenia is related to consumptive coagulopathy that can continue to worsen over several days or if the decrease in platelets is only an acute change due to a single event such as surgery, which is likely to resolve quickly [66]. This approach can help determine the appropriate course of action such as reducing the dose of LMWH by 50% if the platelet count is between 25 and 50×10^9 and cannot be sustained by transfusions or if all anticoagulants should be held with the risk of bleeding exceeding the risk of clotting [47].

4. Adverse effects of anticancer therapy leading to emergent ICU admissions in the adult population

Patients with malignancies are at risk for acute life-threatening illnesses that require intensive care unit (ICU) admission. Leukemia and lymphoma are the most common hematologic cancers encountered in the ICU, and lung cancer is the most common solid tumor encountered in adults [67]. In addition, as many as 40 percent of allogenic hematopoietic cell transplant (HCT) recipients develop one or more complications where transfer to the ICU is necessary [68]. Indications for ICU admission in oncology patients include decompensation secondary to progression of the cancer, treatment-related side effects, or comorbid illnesses.

Patients whose survival rates remain marginally low include allogeneic bone marrow transplant recipients with severe GVHD unresponsive to immunosuppressive therapy, patients with multiple organ failure related to delayed ICU admission, and specific clinical vignettes in patients with solid tumors [69]. They are exposed to individual or combination chemotherapy regimens with the intention of cure or remission but not without risk for developing acute or long-term side effects requiring escalation of care. The following are only a few of the many anticancer therapy-related AEs, and oncology patients may experience resulting in ICU admission.

4.1. Tumor lysis syndrome (TLS)

TLS is an oncologic emergency caused by massive tumor cell lysis with the overwhelming release of intracellular contents (potassium, phosphorus, and nucleic acids) into the systemic circulation. In turn, the kidneys are overwhelmed due to the rapid influx of these contents and inability to excrete them efficiently. This can cause potentially life-threatening metabolic and electrolyte abnormalities which can require a patient to be transferred to an ICU for more appropriate management [70]. The four key electrolyte abnormalities are hyperuricemia (uric acid >8 mg/dL), hyperphosphatemia (phosphate >4.5 mg/dL), hypocalcemia (total serum calcium <7 mg/dL), and hyperkalemia (>6 mmol/L).

TLS manifestations may occur before initiation of chemotherapy but are usually observed within 12–72 h after therapy begins and may persist for 5–7 days post-therapy. TLS occurs most frequently after the initiation of cytotoxic therapy in patients with highly aggressive lymphomas (Burkitt subtype) and acute lymphoblastic leukemia (ALL). TLS may also occur spontaneously and/or in other tumor types that have high proliferation rate, large tumor burden (reflected by serum lactate dehydrogenase levels), or high sensitivity to cytotoxic therapy. Common anticancer agents associated with TLS are listed in **Table 9**.

The Cairo-Bishop grading system is used to classify and grade TLS. TLS is diagnosed by Laboratory Tumor Lysis Syndrome (LTLS) or by Clinical Tumor Lysis Syndrome (CTLS). A retrospective analysis of 772 consecutive acute myeloid leukemia (AML) patients receiving induction chemotherapy concluded clinical TLS (not laboratory) was associated with a significantly higher risk of death during induction therapy (30 out of 38 patients; 79 vs. 23% of those patients without evidence of clinical TLS) [70]. The risk for developing TLS is stratified as low, intermediate, and high risk with treatment strategies varying by each level of risk shown in **Table 10**. Those in the high-risk category strongly need aggressive intervention, and those in the low-risk category might need only observation, but the classification and treatment approach for the intermediate-risk patients is not as clearly defined.

Continuous hydration is the cornerstone of TLS prevention and is recommended prior to therapy in all patients that fall into the intermediate- or high-risk category. The goal is to improve renal perfusion, to improve glomerular filtration rate, and to produce a high urine output to lessen the likelihood of uric acid or calcium phosphate from precipitating in the renal tubules. It is imperative to use cautiously in patients with underlying kidney injury or cardiac dysfunction. The following are key points of this section [72–76]:

- Begin continuous hydration ideally 2 days before chemotherapy is to be given. Continue therapy during chemotherapy administration and 2–3 days after chemotherapy completion. Vigorous hydration (intermediate and high risk) consists of 2–3 L/m^2/day IV solution consisting of 0.225%NS + D5W, with a urine output goal of 80–100 mL/h

- To enhance renal excretion, consider furosemide 20–40 mg IV push to maintain urine output >100 mL/m^2/h or 2 mL/kg/h. Diuretic use is contraindicated if the patient has evidence of acute obstructive uropathy or hypovolemia. Potassium must also be closely monitored due to furosemide's ability to increase renal excretion of this electrolyte.

- The role of urinary alkalization with either acetazolamide and/or sodium bicarbonate is a controversial issue; therefore, use of sodium bicarbonate is only indicated in patients with metabolic acidosis [70].

Bendamustine	Ibrutinib
Bortezomib	Imatinib
Brentuximab Vedotin	Lenalidomide
Carfilzomib	Mechlorethamine
Cetuximab	6-Mercaptopurine
Cisplatin	Nilotinib
Cytarabine	Obinutuzumab
Dasatinib	Omacetaxine
Daunorubicin	Paclitaxel
Doxorubicin	Rituximab
Epirubicin	Romidepsin
Etoposide	Thalidomide
Fludarabine	Vincristine

Table 9. Anticancer agents associated with tumor lysis syndrome (TLS) [71].

Risk category[1]	Treatment options
Low-risk patients	• Observation • Normal hydration with IV fluids • Monitor laboratories once daily throughout chemotherapy, then as clinically indicated post-treatment manage fluid and electrolyte abnormalities • +/− Allopurinol
Intermediate-risk patients	• Vigorous hydration and inpatient monitoring • Initiate allopurinol or rasburicase if uric acid >7.5 mg/dL (Some practices report administering a single dose of rasburicase in this setting, which is a reasonable alternative) • Monitor laboratories every 8–12 h throughout chemotherapy, then as clinically indicated post-treatment • Initiate rasburicase
High-risk patients	• Increase hydration and maintain urine output • Cardiac monitoring • Initiate rasburicase for 1 dose and repeat only if uric acid ≥7.5 mg/dL • Monitor laboratories every 6–8 h throughout chemotherapy, then every 1–2 days post-treatment and as clinically indicated • Manage fluid and electrolyte abnormalities • Consult nephrology
Established TLS in patients	• Admission to Intensive Care Unit • Increase hydration and maintain urine output • Cardiac monitoring • Initiate rasburicase for 1 dose and repeat only if uric acid ≥7.5 mg/dL • At the end of rasburicase treatment, patients should start allopurinol • Monitor laboratories every 4–6 h daily

S/S, signs and symptoms; IVP, intravenous push; CrCl, creatinine clearance; IV, intravenous; NS, normal saline; D5W, 5% dextrose in water; G6PD, glucose-6-phosphate dehydrogenase deficiency; WBC, white blood cells.
[1] Refer to reference [73] for definitions and criteria defining low-, intermediate-, and high-risk patients.

Table 10. Tumor lysis syndrome (TLS) treatment based on risk stratification [72–75].

Allopurinol is a xanthine oxidase inhibitor, which means it blocks the enzyme responsible for the conversion of xanthine to uric acid. Allopurinol is preferred for patients that fall into the low-risk category explained in **Table 10**. It is recommended to start 1–2 days prior to initiating chemotherapy to prevent excess uric acid, but it will not reduce uric acid levels in patients who have existing hyperuricemia [77]. Unfortunately, the excess xanthine levels could precipitate into the kidneys leading to the renal dysfunction. Another limitation of allopurinol is it interferes with the excretion of other chemotherapy agents (high-dose methotrexate, cyclophosphamide, mercaptopurine, and azathioprine). If concomitant use cannot be avoided, reduce 6-mercaptopurine and/or azathioprine doses by 65–75% when used with allopurinol [78]. Allopurinol should never be administered with capecitabine because it may decrease its effectiveness [71]. The recommended oral allopurinol dose per the manufacturer is 600–800 mg daily in divided doses or 100–300 mg oral every 8 h daily (maximum of 800 mg/day). Alternative dosing (off label for intermediate risk for TLS) is 10 mg/kg/day divided every 8 h (maximum of 800 mg per daily) or 50–100 mg/m^2 every 8 h (max dose 300 mg/m^2 daily) beginning 1–2 days before initiation of chemotherapy induction. This may be continue for 3–7 days after chemotherapy [74]. IV allopurinol can be used in patients not tolerating oral at a dose of 200–400 mg/m2/day in one to three divided doses (maximum of 600 mg/day) beginning 1–2 days before initiation of chemotherapy induction and may be continued for 3–7 days after chemotherapy [78]. Allopurinol should be continued until uric acid levels are normalized and tumor burden, WBC count, and other laboratory values have returned to low TLS risk levels as defined in **Table 10**. Refer to **Table 11** for appropriate renal adjustments.

Creatinine Clearance (ml/min)	Daily Oral Allopurinol Dose
Manufacturer Recommended Allopurinol Dosing [78]	
10–20	200 mg
<10	100 mg
<3	100 mg at extended intervals (more than 24 h if necessary)
Alternative Allopurinol Dose Adjustments [74]	
140	400 mg
120	350 mg
100	300 mg
80	250 mg
60	200 mg
40	150 mg
20	100 mg
10	100 mg every 2 days
0	100 mg every 3 days

CrCl, creatinine clearance.

Table 11. Recommended allopurinol dosing.

Rasburicase is a recombinant urate oxidase produced by a genetically modified *S. cerevisiae* strain. Rasburicase is used to treat hyperuricemia by converting uric acid to allantoin thereby reducing uric acid levels and helping to control serum potassium, phosphorus, calcium, and creatinine levels [70]. Allantoin is highly effective with it being five to ten times more soluble in the urine than uric acid. The duration of rasburicase therapy can vary, with a majority receiving 2 days of therapy, but success has been seen with a single dose. Uric acid levels should be monitored regularly and used as a guide for dosing. Rasburicase works quickly with decreases in the level of uric acid by 0.5–1 mg/dL being observed within 4 h of administration [70]. Patients with larger tumor burden may need longer therapy (up to 7 days) or twice daily treatment [70, 78]. Rasburicase is dosed at 0.2 mg/kg/day infused over 30 min with the first dose at least 4 h prior to start of cytotoxic therapy and continued for up to 5 days. Dosing beyond 5 days or administration of more than one course is not recommended [79]. The FDA-approved dose is 0.2 mg/kg dose, but 0.15 mg/kg has demonstrated efficacy, which may be an option for intermediate-risk patients with baseline uric acid ≤7.5 mg/dL [70]. Many institutions are also utilizing fixed dosages (3, 6 or 7.5 mg) versus weight based dosing [97]. Once serum uric acid levels normalize, rasburicase can be stopped and allopurinol treatment can be initiated/resumed. Concomitant allopurinol should not be administered in order to avoid xanthine accumulation and lack of substrate for rasburicase.

4.2. Pulmonary complications (non-infectious causes) following hematopoietic stem cell transplantation (HCT)

Hematopoietic stem cell transplantation (HCT) is a treatment option for many malignant hematological disorders. The conditioning chemotherapy regimens used are considered either myeloablative where lethal doses of chemotherapy are given, with or without irradiation, or non-myeloablative where lower doses of chemotherapy are administered. Our lungs contain an enormous capillary bed that is uniquely sensitive to the side effects of chemotherapy and radiation therapy. Subsequently, a myeloablative conditioning regimen with lethal doses of chemotherapy has a high likelihood of causing pulmonary complications. The estimated incidence of pulmonary complications in HCT recipients ranges between 40 and 60% [80]. Such complications can be further divided into infectious and non-infectious causes. The non-infectious causes include pulmonary edema, engraftment syndrome (ES), diffuse alveolar hemorrhage (DAH), idiopathic pneumonia syndrome (IPS), bronchiolitis obliterans organizing pneumonia (BOOP), and pulmonary sarcoidosis. The risk of developing these complications can occur at three different phases following a HCT. The neutropenic phase is described as <30 days post-HCT, the early phase includes 30–100 days post-HCT, and the late phase is known as >100 days post-HCT. The following section will focus on a few of the non-infectious pulmonary complications that occur in the neutropenic phase (<30 days) post-HCT.

Engraftment syndrome is equally common in autologous and allogenic HCT patients (7–11 and 10%, respectively). The median time to onset is 10 days post-transplant and can manifest up to 11 days. The syndrome is multifactorial consisting of the overproduction and release of pro-inflammatory cytokines and interaction between T cells, monocytes, and complement activation during engraftment. A majority of the cases are mild and self-limiting but the moderate-to-severe cases require treatment with corticosteroids. Lack of response to corticosteroid therapy leading to mechanical ventilation is a predictor of poor prognosis [76].

Treatment for mild ES (transient low-grade fevers with limited rash) includes discontinuing G-CSF and initiating empiric broad-spectrum antibiotics. Moderate-to-severe ES with pulmonary involvement often requires treatment with corticosteroids such as methylprednisolone doses ranging from 0.5 to 10 mg/kg/day or methylprednisolone 1–2 g/day × 3 days followed by rapid taper over 2–3 weeks. A decrease in O_2 requirement should be observed with symptoms improving in 2–4 days [13, 81, 82].

Diffuse alveolar hemorrhage (DAH) is a progressive, non-infectious pulmonary complication following HCT often leading to mechanical ventilation for respiratory failure in a majority of patients. It is thought to be due to a combination of mechanisms such as lung tissue injury from the conditioning regimen or pulmonary infections, inflammation likely due to a combination of bronchial inflammation, alveolitis, GCSF induced neutrophil influx into the lungs, or cytokine release which contributes to alveolar capillary endothelial membrane damage. DAH occurs equally in approximately 5% of allogeneic and autologous HCT recipients with the most common cause of death being multi-organ failure and sepsis [76, 83–85]. Standard therapy includes high-dose corticosteroids with methylprednisolone 500–1000 mg/day for 3–4 days followed by 1 mg/kg for 3 days then taper over 2–4 weeks. Doses of 125–250 mg IV every 6 h for the first 4–5 days followed by a taper over 2–4 weeks have been associated with higher overall survival as well. One retrospective study of 14 patients also showed an overall higher survival benefit with aminocaproic acid 1000 mg IV q6 h plus methylprednisolone 250 mg IV every 6 h followed by a taper. In addition, several case reports have shown a modest resolution in bleeding with the combination of recombinant factor VIIa 90 mcg/kg and methylprednisolone 500–2000 mg IV daily followed by gradual taper over 2–4 weeks [76, 84–86].

4.3. Cytokine release syndrome (CRS) associated with chimeric antigen receptors (CARs)

Immunotherapy is redefining the standard of care in many malignancies. Recent advances involve the engineering of a patient's own immune cells to recognize and attack tumor cells. T cells contain a monoclonal antibody fragment (scFv) specific for a tumor target with T-cell receptor activation. The T cells are then directed to target antigens that are expressed by tumors. This initiates the patient's own immune system to target the cancer. However, CAR T-cell treatments are not without risks, and many people experience an inflammatory process called severe cytokine release syndrome (CRS) that requires hospitalization, with over 30% requiring intensive care admission [87].

Cytokine release syndrome (CRS) is marked by dramatic elevation in cytokine levels producing a systemic inflammatory response similar to that of septic shock. The onset has been noted to occur within 1–14 days of CD-19 CAR T-cell infusion and resolves typically in 2–3 weeks. With hypotension being the main criteria in the revised CRS grading system, it is important to record baseline blood pressure prior to start of therapy that could induce CRS. Potentially life-threatening complications with CRS include cardiac dysfunction, adult respiratory distress syndrome, neurologic toxicity, renal failure, hepatic failure, and disseminated intravascular coagulation [85]. Diagnosis of CRS is made based on the presence of high levels of inflammatory markers and cytokines, increased LFTs, and increased total bilirubin [88]. Appropriate treatment is based on the CRS grading system explained in **Table 12**.

CRS-revised grading system	Treatment Associated with revised grading system
Grade 1 Symptoms are not life threatening and require symptomatic treatment only: Fever and constitutional symptoms (nausea, fatigue, headache, myalgias, malaise)	• Assess for infection in all grades • Vigilant supportive care including antipyretics and analgesics in all grades[1]
Grade 2 Symptoms require and respond to moderate intervention Oxygen requirement <40% or Hypotension responsive to fluids or Vasopressor if unresponsive to fluids or Grade 2 organ toxicity	• Monitor cardiac function (s/s cardiac decomposition). Cardiac decompensation can be sudden and severe, but usually reversible. The pathophysiology of acute cardiac toxicity in the setting of CRS is not clear, but resembles cardiomyopathy associated with sepsis and stress cardiomyopathy. Monitor echocardiography frequently in patients who are a concern for cardiac dysfunction (Grade 2–4) • Monitor organ function closely • Monitor/manage complications of TLS IF, older age or extensive comorbidities: • Based on clinical judgment, may be necessary to initiate immunosuppressive therapy (refer to Grade 3/4 treatment)
Grade 3 Symptoms require and respond to aggressive intervention Oxygen requirement ≥40% or Hypotension requiring high dose or multiple vasopressors or Grade 3 organ toxicity or grade 4 transaminitis	• Initiate **tocilizumab**: For patients weighing <30 kg: 12 mg/kg IV x1 dose For patients weighing >30 kg: 8 mg/kg IV × 1 dose (max dose 800 mg)
Grade 4 Life-threatening symptoms Requirement for ventilator support or Grade 4 organ toxicity (excluding transaminitis)	IF, lack of clinical improvement while waiting for tocilizumab response: • Initiate corticosteroid therapy (taper within one week; can generally be accomplished) **Methylprednisolone**[*] 2mg/kg x 1 dose, followed by 2mg/kg/d divided 4 times per day [24] to hopefully suppress the inflammatory cascade and prevent irreversible organ dysfunction
Grade 5—Death	

[*]Emerging evidence suggests corticosteroids may mediate a greater adverse effect on the antitumor activity of adoptively transferred T cells [26]

[1] Vigilant supportive care: antipyretics, analgesics, adequate hydration, blood pressure support, and broad-spectrum antibiotics.

[2] For patients with severe neurologic symptoms, consider dexamethasone (0.5 mg/kg; maximum 10 mg/dose) due to more efficient penetration of the blood-brain barrier although evidence for choosing one over the other has not been established.

Table 12. Cytokine release syndrome–revised grading system and associated treatment [88–90].

Tocilizumab is an antirheumatic disease modifying interleukin-6 receptor antagonist approved for adults with rheumatoid arthritis at the dose 4–8 mg/kg every 4 weeks infused over 1 h [88]. It is also the standard therapy for managing Grade 3 CRS. Reports have shown cytokines return to normal and symptoms resolve concurrently by day nine following tocilizumab administration [87, 91]. In addition, tocilizumab may have less impact on the antitumor effect of CAR t cells when compared to corticosteroids [88]. If the patient has a positive clinical response to tocilizumab, then vasopressors and supportive measures can be weaned shortly thereafter. If the patient's condition does not improve or stabilize within 24 h of tocilizumab dose, a second dose can be administered. A corticosteroid regimen should also be considered if it has not already been initiated. Adverse effects (AE) associated with tocilizumab include, but are not limited to: hypersensitivity reactions, elevated liver enzymes, fatal opportunistic infections, gastrointestinal perforation, hematologic effects, herpes zoster reactivation, hyperlipidemia, and tuberculosis. Studies are under investigation regarding the optimal timing of anti-Il-6 treatment, but some levels of CRS should be expected and possibly an inevitable consequence of the CAR T-cell therapy mechanism [92].

4.4. Pulmonary toxicity due to chemotherapy agents in general oncology patients

In the non-HCT patients, several other chemotherapy agents have high risks for causing pulmonary toxicity exhibited early with infiltrates, pulmonary edema, hypersensitivity reactions, and pleural effusions or with infiltrates or fibrosis in late onset (greater than 2 months). These injuries can be dose dependent or can manifest several years after completion of therapy [93]. As a result, the most severe and late stages of such toxicity are usually observed in patients admitted to the ICU. The most common chemotherapy agents associated with pulmonary toxicity and their respective clinical/radiologic manifestations are described in **Table 13**. The mainstay treatment for such pulmonary complications are largely steroids; however, it has yet to be determined the appropriate dose and duration of therapy that is most effective. One study evaluated the dosage pattern of corticosteroids used in 398 lung cancer patients with pulmonary toxicity. The drug-induced interstitial lung diseases were primarily treated with pulse dose therapy (≥500 mg/day methylprednisolone for 3 days followed by high-dose steroids) and high-dose therapy (≥0.5 mg/kg/day prednisolone). These cases had a mortality rate of 48.4% which was similar or less than that of the other groups. Unfortunately, response to therapy was not defined in this study by improvements in radiologic findings or carbon monoxide diffusing capacity, which has been suggested as better indicators [94]. Scarce literature exists outside of case series or small observation studies as the one described. Therefore, with the lack of established treatment guidelines for pulmonary toxicity, intensivists should customize corticosteroid regimens based on each patient's response and risk for AEs from prolonged therapy.

Despite the many advances in cancer treatment options including not only chemotherapy but also immunotherapy agents, the risks for AEs have unfortunately not been completely diminished. These agents are administered at toxic levels with multiple cycles, and each dose highly affects more than one organ system. Therefore, the risks observed from these agents far outweigh AEs due to therapies initiated in typical ICU patients. The AEs previously discussed are only a few of the many acute and chronic consequences that are observed in cancer patients leading to ICU admission. However, the pharmacologic management of such occurrences is extremely important as they affect future treatment options and overall quality of life of the patient.

Chemotherapy agent	Clinical/radiological manifestations
Bleomycin	Bronchiolitis obliterans organizing pneumonia (now referred to as *cryptogenic organizing pneumonia*), eosinophilic hypersensitivity, or interstitial pneumonitis (most common) that can progress to fibrosis
Methotrexate	Bilateral interstitial and alveolar infiltrates or pleural effusions, accompanied by fever and peripheral eosinophilia. Fibrosis can be prevented if the medication is discontinued
Gemcitabine	Diffuse ground-glass changes accompanied by thickened septal lines, interstitial infiltrates, or diffuse alveolar infiltrates, which may lead to acute respiratory distress syndrome
Paclitaxel	Bilateral reticular or ground-glass infiltrates or focal consolidation
Oxaliplatin	Interstitial pneumonitis with fibrosis occurring after 3–6 months of therapy. Patients can present with slow progressive cough and dyspnea
EGFR-targeted inhibitors: gefitinib and erlotinib	Airspace consolidation or extensive bilateral ground-glass infiltrates

Table 13. Common chemotherapy agents associated with pulmonary toxicity and clinical/radiological manifestations [005B93].

Author details

Trisha Patel*, Erica M. McGovern, Denise Wolfe, Mark E. Lewis and Mashiul Chowdhury

*Address all correspondence to: trisha.patel@ctca-hope.com

Cancer Treatment Centers of America at Eastern Regional Medical Center, Philadelphia, USA

References

[1] Thirumala R, Ramaswany M, Chawla S. Diagnosis and management of infectious complications in critically-ill patients with cancer. Crit Care Clin. 2010; 26: 59–91.

[2] Portillo ME, Corvec S, et al. *Propionibacterium acnes:* an underestimated pathogen in implant-associated infections. BioMed Res Int. 2013; 2013. Article ID: 804391: 1–10.

[3] Pruitt A, David Schiff, Santosh Kesari, Patrick Y Wen. Central nervous system infections in cancer patients. In: Current Clinical Oncology. Neurological Complications of Cancer and Its Treatment, 2nd ed. Totowa: Humana Press; 2008: 354–379.

[4] Tunkel AR, Harman BJ, et al. Practice guidelines for the management of bacterial meningitis. Clin Infect Dis. 2004; 39: 1267–1284.

[5] Homsi J, Walsh D, et al. Infectious complications of advanced cancer. Support Care Cancer. 2000; 8: 487–492.

[6] Paick SH, Park HK, et al. Characteristics of bacterial colonization and urinary tract infection after indwelling of double-J ureteral stent. Urology. 2003; 62: 214–217.

[7] Hooton TM, Bradley SF, et al. Diagnosis, prevention, and treatment of catheter-associated urinary tract infection in adults: 2009 international clinical practice guidelines from the Infectious Diseases Society of America. Clin Infect Dis. 2010; 50: 625–663.

[8] Kim-Hsu C, Hoag JB, et al. The microbiology of post obstructive pneumonia in lung cancer patients. J Bronchol Intervent Pulmonol. 2013; 20: 266–270.

[9] Toussiant E, Bahel-Ball E, et al. Causes of fever in cancer patients (prospective study over 477 episodes). Support Care Cancer. 2006; 14: 763–769.

[10] Marinella M. Fever in patients with cancer. In: Yu V, Burdette S, editors. Antimicrobial Therapy and Vaccines: Empiric. Antimicrobe. Infectious Disease and Antimicrobial Agents. E-Sun Technologies. Available at: http://www.antimicrobe.org/e13.asp

[11] Shomali W, Hachem R, et al. Can procalcitonin distinguish infectious fever from tumor-related fever in non-neutropenic cancer patients? Cancer. 2012; 118: 5823–5829.

[12] O'Grady NP, Barie PS, et al. Guidelines for evaluation of new fever in critically ill adult patients: 2008 update from the American College of Critical Care Medicine and the Infectious Diseases Society of America. Crit Care Med. 2008; 36: 1330–1349.

[13] Rybak M, Lomaestro B, et al. Therapeutic monitoring of vancomycin in adult patients: a consensus review of the American Society of Health-System Pharmacists, the Infectious Diseases Society of America, and the Society of Infectious Diseases Pharmacists. Am J Health Syst Pharm. 2009; 66: 82–98.

[14] Al-Kofide H, Zaghloul I, Al-Naim L. Pharmacokinetics of vancomycin in adult cancer patients. J Oncol Pharm Practice. 2010; 16: 245–250.

[15] Prybylski JP. Vancomycin trough concentration as a predictor of clinical outcomes in patients with *Staphylococcus aureus* bacteremia: a meta-analysis of observation studies. Pharmacotherapy. 2015; 35 (10): 889–898.

[16] Pea F, Poz D, et al. Optimisation of vancomycin regimen in neutropenic haematoligcal patients with normal renal function. Multiple daily doses may be preferable. Clin Drug Invest Mar. 2000; 19 (3): 213–218.

[17] Blot SI, Pea F, Lipman J. The effect of pathophysiology on pharmacokinetics in the critically ill patient—concepts appraised by the example of antimicrobial agents. Adv Drug Deliv Rev. 2014; 77: 3–11.

[18] Lodise TP, Lomaesstro B., et al. Piperacillin-tazobactam for *Pseudomonas aeruginosa* infection: clinical implications of an extended-infusion dosing strategy. Clin Infect Dis. 2007; 44: 357–363.

[19] Dow RJ, Rose WE, et al. Retrospective study of prolonged versus intermittent infusion Piperacillin-tazobactam and meropenem in intensive care unit patients at an Academic Medical Center. Infect Dis Clin Pract. 2011; 19 (6): 413–417.

[20] Chant C, Leung A, et al. Optimal dosing of antibiotics in critically-ill patients using continuous/extended infusions: a systematic review and meta-analysis. Crit Care. 2013; 17: R279.

[21] Rhodes NJ, MacVane SH, et al. Impact of loading doses on the time to adequate predicted beta-lactam concentrations in prolonged and continuous infusion dosing schemes. Correspondence. Clin Infect Dis. 2014; 59: 905–907.

[22] Patel N, Scheetz MH, et al. Identification of optimal renal dosage adjustments for traditional and extended-infusion Piperacillin-tazobactam dosing regimens in hospitalized patients. Antimicrob Agents Chemother. 2010; 54 (1): 460–465.

[23] Feher C, Rovira M, et al. Effect of meropenem administration in extended infusion on the clinical outcome of febrile neutropenia: a retrospective observational study. J Antimicrob Chemother. 2014; 69: 2556–2562.

[24] Mattoes HM, Kuti JL, et al. Optimizing antimicrobial pharmacodynamics: dosage strategies for meropenem. Clin Ther. 2004; 26 (8): 1187–1198.

[25] Carlier M, Carrette S, et al. Meropenem and piperacillin-tazobactam prescribing in critically-ill patients: does augmented renal clearance affect pharmacokinetic/pharmacodynamics target attainment when extended infusions are used? Crit Care. 2013; 17: R84.

[26] Antibiotic Resistant Threats in the United States. U.S. Department of Health and Human Services. Centers for Disease Control and Prevention, 2013. http://www.cdc.gov/drugresistance/threat-report-2013/pdf/ar-threats-2013-508.pdf.

[27] Kaye KS, Pogue JM. Infections caused by resistant gram-negative bacteria: epidemology and management. Pharmacotherapy. 2015; 35 (10): 949–962.

[28] AVYCAZ (ceftazidime and avibactam) [package insert]. Verona, Italy: GlaxoSmithKline; 2015.

[29] Giamarellou H, Galani L, et al. Effectiveness of double-carbapenem regimen for infections in humans due to carbapenemase-producing pan-drug resistant *Klebsiella pneumoniae*. Antimicrob Agents Chemother. 2013; 57 (5): 2388–2390.

[30] Bulick CC, Nicolau DP. Double-carbapenem therapy for carbapenemase-producing klebsiella pneumoniae. Antimicrob Agents Chemother. 2011; 55 (6): 3002–3004.

[31] Yamamoto M, Pop-Vicas AE. Treatment of infections with carbapenem-resistant *Enterobacteriaceae*: what options do we still have? Crit Care. 2014; 18: 229.

[32] Akajabor DS, Wilson SL, et al. Higher incidence of acute kidney injury with intravenous colistimethate sodium compared with polymixin B in critically-ill patients at a Tertiary Care Medical Center. Clin Infect Dis. 2013; 57 (9): 1300–1303.

[33] Morrill HJ, Pogue JM, et al. Treatment options for carbapenem-resistant enterobacteriaceae infections. Open Forum Infect Dis. 2015; 2(2):ofv050. doi: 10.1093/ofid/ofv050.

[34] Kanj SS, Kanafani ZA. Current concepts in antimicrobial therapy against resistant gram-negative organisms: extended-spectrum β-lactamase-producing enterobacteriaceae, carbapenem-resistant enterobacteriaceae, and multi-drug resistant *Pseudomonas aeruginosa*. Mayo Clin Proc. 2011; 86(3): 250–259.

[35] Zasowski EJ, Rybak JM, Rybak MJ. The b-Lactams Strike Back: Ceftazidime-Avibactam. *Pharmacotherapy* 2015;35(8):755–770) doi: 10.1002/phar.1622.

[36] ZERBAXA (ceftolozane and tazobactam) [package insert]. Syracuse, NY: Merck & Co; 2015.

[37] Cohen SH, Gerding DN, et al. Clinical practice guidelines for clostridium difficile infection in adults: 2010 update by the Society for Healthcare Epidemiology of America (SHEA) and the Infectious Diseases Society of America (IDSA). Infect Control Hosp Epidemiol. 2010; 31 (5): 431–455.

[38] Rokas KEE, Johnson JW, et al. The addition of intravenous metronidazole to oral vancomycin is associated with improved mortality in critically-ill patients with clostridium difficile infection. Clin Infect Dis. 2015; 61(6): 934–941.

[39] Doron S, Snydman DR. Risk and safety of probiotics. Clin Infect Dis. 2015; 60 (S2): S129–S134.

[40] Podnos YD, Jimenez JC, Wilson SE. Intra-abdominal sepsis in elderly persons. Clin Infect Dis. 2002; 35: 62–68.

[41] Anaya DA, Dellinger EP. Necrotizing soft-tissue infection: diagnosis and management. Clin Infect Dis. 2007; 44 (5): 705–710.

[42] Foo RM, Tung ML, et al. Necrotizing fasciitis in hematological patients: Enterobacteriaceae Predominance and Limited Utility of Laboratory risk indicator for necrotizing fasciitis score. Open Forum Infect Dis. 2015; 2(2): OFID: 1–4.

[43] Blank M, Chowdhury M. *Stenotrophomonas maltophilia* infection in a febrile neutropenia patient. Infect Med. 2006; 23: 130–132.

[44] Stevens DL, Bisno AL, et al. Practice guidelines for the diagnosis and management of skin and soft tissue infections: 2014 update by the Infectious Diseases Society of America. IDSA practice guidelines for SSTIs. Clin Infect Dis. 2014; 59 (2): e10–e52.

[45] Al-Niaimi F, Cox N. Cellulitis and lymphoedema: a viscious cycle. J Lymphoedema. 2009; 4 (2): 38–42.

[46] Kourlaba G, Relakis J, Kontodimas S, Holm M, Maniadakis N. The humanistic and economic burden of venous thromboembolism in cancer patients: a systematic review. Value Health. 2013; 16 (7): A403–A404. doi:10.1016/j.jval.2013.08.465.

[47] Watson H, Keeling D, Laffan M, Tait R, Makris M. Guideline on aspects of cancer-related venous thrombosis. Br J Haematol. 2015; 170 (5): 640–648. doi:10.1111/bjh.13556.

[48] Timp J, Braekkan S, Versteeg H, Cannegieter S. Epidemiology of cancer-associated venous thrombosis. Blood. 2013; 122 (10): 1712–1723. doi:10.1182/blood-2013-04-460121.

[49] Wun T, White R. Epidemiology of cancer-related venous thromboembolism. Best Pract Res Clin Haematol. 2009; 22 (1): 9–23. doi:10.1016/j.beha.2008.12.001.

[50] Chan M, Shorr AF. Venous thromboembolic disease in the intensive care unit. Semin Respir Crit Care Med. 2010; 31 (1): 39–46.

[51] Cook D, Crowther M, et al. Deep venous thrombosis in medical-surgical critically ill patients: prevalence, incidence, and risk factors. Crit Care Med. 2005; 33: 1565–1571.

[52] Debourdeau P, Farge D, Beckers M, et al. International clinical practice guidelines for the treatment and prophylaxis of thrombosis associated with central venous catheters in patients with cancer. J Thromb Haemostasis. 2013; 11 (1): 71–80. doi:10.1111/jth.12071.

[53] Lyman G, Bohlke K, Falanga A. Venous thromboembolism prophylaxis and treatment in patients with cancer: American Society of Clinical Oncology clinical practice guideline update. J Oncol Pract. 2015; 11 (3): e442–e444. doi:10.1200/jop.2015.004473.

[54] NCCN Clinical Practice Guidelines in Oncology. Cancer-associated venous thromboembolic disease, 2015. Available at: http://www.nccn.org/professionals/physician_gls/pdf/vte.pdf (accessed January 2, 2016).

[55] Kahn SR, Lim W, et al. Prevention of VTE in Nonsurgical Patients Antithrombotic Therapy and Prevention of Thrombosis, 9th ed. American College of Chest Physicians Evidence-Based Clinical Practice Guidelines. Chest. 2012; 141 (Suppl. 2): e195S–e226S.

[56] Gould MK, Garcia DA, et al. Prevention of VTE in Nonorthopedic Surgical Patients Antithrombotic Therapy and Prevention of Thrombosis, 9th ed. American College of chest physicians evidence-based clinical practice guidelines. Chest. 2012; 141 (Suppl. 2): e227S–e277S.

[57] Kearon C, Akl EA, et al. Antithrombotic Therapy for VTE Disease Antithrombotic Therapy and Prevention of Thrombosis, 9th ed. American College of chest physicians evidence-based clinical practice guidelines. Chest. 2012; 141 (Suppl. 2): e419S–e494S.

[58] Kakkos SK, Caprini JA, Geroulakos G, et al. Combined intermittent pneumatic leg compression and pharmacological prophylaxis for prevention of venous thromboembolism in high-risk patients. Cochrane Database Syst Rev. 2008; 4: CD005258.

[59] Ageno W, Gallus A, Wittkowsky A, Crowther M, Hylek E, Palareti G. Oral anticoagulant therapy. Chest. 2015; 141 (2): e44S–e88S.

[60] Sholzberg M, Pavenski K, Shehata N, Cserti-Gazdewich C, Lin Y. Bleeding complications from the direct oral anticoagulants. BMC Hematol. 2015; 15:1–5. doi:10.1186/s12878-015-0039-z.

[61] Thaler J, Pabinger I, Ay C. Anticoagulant treatment of deep vein thrombosis and pulmonary embolism: the present state of the art. Front Cardiovasc Med. 2015; 2(30): 1–7. doi:10.3389/fcvm.2015.00030.

[62] Weitz J. New antithrombotic drugs. Chest. 2012; 141 (Suppl. 2): e120S. doi:10.1378/chest.11-2294.

[63] Xarelto [package insert]. Titusville, NJ: Janssen; 2012.

[64] Apixaban Medical Information. Bristol: Myers Squibb; 2015.

[65] Mantha S, Ansell J. Indirect comparison of dabigatran, rivaroxaban, apixaban and edoxaban for the treatment of acute venous thromboembolism. J Thromb Thrombol. 2014; 39 (2): 155–165. doi:10.1007/s11239-014-1102-5.

[66] Greinacher A, Selleng K. Thrombocytopenia in the intensive care unit patient. ASH Educ Book. 2010; 2010 (1): 135–143.

[67] Kress JP, Christenson J, Pohlman AS, et al. Outcomes of critically-ill cancer patients in a university hospital setting. Am J Respir Crit Care Med. 1999; 160: 1957.

[68] Freedman N, Hansen-Flaschen J. Prognosis of cancer patients in the intensive care unit. Updated: Oct. 2015. (accessed December 29, 2015) http://www.uptodate.com/contents/prognosis-of-cancer-patients-in-the-intensive-care-unit?source=search_result search=prognosis+of+cancer+patients+in+the+intensive+care+unit selectedTitle=1%7E150.

[69] Azoulay E, et al. Intensive care of the cancer patient: recent achievements and remaining challenges. Ann Intensive Care. 2011; 1: 5.

[70] Larson R, Pui C. Tumor lysis syndrome: prevention and treatment. Updated: April 2013. (accessed December 29, 2015) http://www.uptodate.com/contents/tumor-lysis-syndrome-prevention-and-treatment?source=search_result search=tumor+lysis+syndrome+prevention+and+treatment selectedTitle=1%7E150.

[71] Held-Warmkessel J. Preventing and managing tumor lysis syndrome. Oncol Times. 2010; 32 (8): 1–7.

[72] Allen A, Mekoba B. Oncologic emergencies: hypercalcemia of malignancy and tumor lysis syndrome. U.S. Pharmacist Supplement. 2015; 40(5): 3–7.

[73] The University of Texas MD Anderson Cancer Center. Tumor lysis in adult Patients algorithm. 2013. Available at: https://www.mdanderson.org/education-and-researcha (accessed January 31, 2016).

[74] Coiffier B, Altman A, Pui CH, et al. Guidelines for the management of pediatric and adult tumor lysis syndrome: an evidence based review. J Clin Oncol. 2008; 26: 2767.

[75] Boyiadzis M, et al. Hematology-Oncology Therapy, 2nd ed. United States: McGraw-Hill Education; 2014. Print.

[76] Ganetsky A. Non-infectious pulmonary complications in hematopoietic stem cell transplantation. In: NMDP Recommended Guidelines. Be the Match Conference Handouts. Hematology Oncology Pharmacist Association (HOPA). Austin TX; 2015.

[77] Trinh, V. 2015. NCCN Immuno-Oncology Webinar Series for Pharmacists; Part 3. Identification and Management of Toxicities with Immuno-oncologic Therapy; 2015 https://education.nccn.org/node/73752.

[78] Allopurinol (Zyloprim®) package insert. Manufactured by DSM Pharmaceuticals, Inc. San Diego, CA; 2003.

[79] Rasburicase Drug Information. In: Micromedex® Solutions. Ann Arbor, MI: Truven Health Analytics. Available at: www.micromedexsolutions.com (accessed February 8, 2016).

[80] Benz R, Schanz U, Maggiorini M, et al. Risk factors for ICU admission and ICU survival after allogenic hematopoietic SCT. Bone Marrow Transplant. 2014; 49: 62.

[81] Maiolino A, Biasoli I, Lima J, Portugal AC, Pulcheri W, Nucci M. Engraftment syndrome following autologous hematopoietic stem cell transplantation: definition of diagnostic criteria. Bone Marrow Transplant. 2001; 27: 393–397.

[82] Clark JG, Hansen JA, Hertz MI, Parkman R, Jensen L, Peavy HH. NHLBI workshop summary. Idiopathic pneumonia syndrome after bone marrow transplantation. Am Rev Respir Dis. 1993; 147: 1601–1605.

[83] Afessa B, Tefferi A, Litzow M, Krowka MJ, Wylam ME, Peters SG. Diffuse alveolar hemorrhage in hematopoietic stem cell transplant recipients. Am J Respir Crit Care Med. 2002; 166: 641–645.

[84] Metcalf JP, Rennard SI, Reed EC, et al. Corticosteroids as adjunctive therapy for diffuse alveolar haemorrhage associated with bone marrow transplantation. University of Nebraska Medical Center Bone Marrow Transplant Group. Am J Med. 1994; 96: 327–334.

[85] Heslet L, Nielsen JD, Levi M, Sengelov H, Johansson PI. Successful pulmonary administration of activated recombinant factor VII in diffuse alveolar hemorrhage. Crit Care. 2006; 10: R177.

[86] Majhail NS, Schiffer CA, Weisdorf DJ. Improvement in pulmonary function with imatinib mesylate in bronchiolitis obliterans following allogenic hematopoietic cell transplantation. Biol Blood Marrow Transplant. 2006; 12: 789–791.

[87] Weiner GJ. Rituximab: mechanism of action. Semin Hematol. 2010; 47 (2): 115–123.

[88] Lee D, Gardner R, Porter D, et al. Current concepts in the diagnosis and management of cytokine release syndrome. Blood. 2014; 124 (2): 188–195.

[89] Singh K, Carson K, Shah R, et al. Meta-analysis of clinical correlates of acute mortality in takotsubo cardiomyopathy. Am J Cardiol. 2014; 113 (8): 1420–1428.

[90] Tocilizumab Drug Information. In: Micromedex® Solutions. Ann Arbor, MI: Truven Health Analytics. Available at: www.micromedexsolutions.com (accessed January 21, 2016).

[91] Harris T, Drake C. Primer on tumor immunology and cancer immunotherapy. J Immuno Ther Cancer. 2013; 1: 12.

[92] Louis C, Savoldo B, et al. Antitumor activity and long term fate of chimeric antigen receptor-positive T cells in patients with neuroblastoma. Blood. 2011; 118: 6050–6056.

[93] Torrisi JM, Schwartz LH, et al. CT Findings of chemotherapy-induced toxicity. Radiology. 2011; 258 (1): 41–56.

[94] Kim S, Oh I, et al. Corticosteroid therapy against treatment-related pulmonary toxicities in patients with lung cancer. J Thorac Dis. 2014; 6 (9): 1209–1217.

[95] Chopra T, Alangaden GJ, Chandrasekar P. Clostridium difficile infection in cancer patients and hematopoietic stem cell transplant recipients. Expert Rev of Anti-infective Ther. 2010; 8 (10): 1113.

[96] Nation RL, Garonzik SM, et al. Updated US and European dose recommendations for intravenous colistin: how do they perform? Clin Infect Dis. 2016; 62(5): 552–558.

[97] Allopurinol drug information: In: Micromedex®Solutions [www.micromedexsolutions.com] Ann Arbor (MI): Truven Health Analytics (Accessed 2016-02-08).

Chapter 3

Improving Outcome in Gastrointestinal and Hepatopancreaticobiliary Surgical Oncology by Preoperative Risk Assessment and Optimization of Perioperative Care

Audrey C.H.M. Jongen, Victor van Woerden,
Jeroen L.A. van Vugt, Patrick A. de Hoogt,
Elisabeth M.L. de Wijkerslooth de Weerdesteijn,
Juul J.W. Tegels, Nicole D. Bouvy and
Jan H.M.B. Stoot

Additional information is available at the end of the chapter

http://dx.doi.org/10.5772/64775

Abstract

This chapter discusses the most important challenges in the perioperative phase of the oncology patient undergoing surgery of the gastrointestinal tract. Because of the aging population, the surgeon is ever more confronted with frail patients at risk for an adverse surgical outcome. The chapter therefore reviews factors contributing to an impaired postoperative outcome such as sarcopenia, frailty, cachexia, and malnutrition and gives an insight into their pathophysiology. Next, it provides an overview of validated preoperative classification systems to identify the patients at risk for surgical complications. Furthermore, it discusses the most essential recommendations of standardized care for patients undergoing hepatopancreaticobiliary, gastric, and colorectal surgery. Special attention is paid to the use of clinical pathways in the perioperative phase that are aimed at a multimodal approach of reducing surgical morbidity by lowering the perioperative physiological and psychological stress. Recent literature is discussed regarding care in the intensive care unit, and the final paragraph focuses on improving postoperative outcome by means of prehabilitation or exercise as well as dietary interventions and optimized nutrition.

Keywords: surgical oncology, risk assessment, frailty, sarcopenia, cachexia, clinical pathways, prehabilitation, dietary interventions

1. Introduction in surgical oncology of the abdomen

1.1. General introduction

Cancers of the gastrointestinal (GI) and hepatopancreaticobiliary (HPB) tract entail some of the most prevalent, as well as some of the most lethal, cancers worldwide [1]. Surgery for cancer of the digestive tract involves extensive and complex procedures and is associated with high complication rates [2]. In the past decades, however, the clinical outcome of patients undergoing surgery for gastrointestinal malignancies has improved significantly. Besides the changes in surgical technique, such as the introduction of minimally invasive surgery and the implementation of novel medical devices, the anesthetic and perioperative care have also evolved [3]. Patients operated with laparoscopic techniques showed a reduction in various inflammatory responses and improved immune function when compared to patients undergoing open surgery in several randomized clinical trials. These studies, however, did not take into account the change in perioperative care that was brought about by the faster recovery following laparoscopic surgery. More recent randomized controlled trials standardized care for both arms and found better outcomes for patients treated with laparoscopy and clinical care pathways, in most [4, 5], but not in all cases [6].

Many important factors have been described that influence the surgical outcome of the surgical oncology patient population. These factors are present in a wide range of surgical patients, but particularly high rates have been described in the elderly population. Aging is accompanied by high prevalence of comorbidities and a decreased functional reserve, all of which can contribute to an increased risk for complications such as delirium, pressure ulcers, infection, functional decline, and other surgery-specific complications. While the increased quality of care is advantageous for the general oncological population, improvement in outcome for elderly patients has remained relatively limited [7, 8]. This is a worrisome fact, as the aging Western population leads to an increase of elderly people diagnosed with cancer and, consequently, more elderly people in need of surgical care. Many of the currently available treatment guidelines for surgical oncology patients are based on clinical data from a patient population with a relative low number of old and more frail patients. Therefore, in order to further improve outcomes also for our most vulnerable patients, identifying those at highest risk of poor outcome is of paramount importance.

The need for tools that provide insight in our patients' health status prior to undergoing surgery has become overt. It has been shown that functional compromise, defined by several conditions such as fatigue, sarcopenia, cachexia, malnutrition, vulnerability, and frailty, has a major impact on the risk of the development of complications and on postoperative outcome

http://dx.doi.org/10.5772/64775

in general. These conditions show strong overlap in several clinical features, which make strict separation of these syndromes rather difficult.

Several authors have described questionnaires and tests that allow surgeons to identify the patients at high risk. With these tools, patients that are prone to developing complications can be selected for a broad range of intervention types that are aimed at optimizing the condition of the surgical patient and consequently to improve postoperative outcome. To date, a wide variety of validated risk assessment tools have been described. Some of those have already successfully been introduced into clinical practice, such as the ASA (American Society of Anesthesiologist) classification, the Surgical Outcome Risk Tool (SORT) [9], and the Surgical Risk Calculator from the American College of Surgeons [10]. Many other, more specific scoring systems or tests have been designed to assess frailty (Comprehensive Geriatric Assessment [11], Fried Frailty Phenotype [12], timed "up and go" test [13], Groningen Frailty Index [14]), or nutritional state (Short Nutritional Assessment Questionnaire (SNAQ) [15], Malnutrition Universal Screening Tool (MUST)) [12, 16]. These assessment tools are designed to identify the patients at high risk for perioperative complications and adverse outcomes. Moreover, these may help the physician in the selection of patients that may benefit from "prehabilitation" and nutritional and other interventions.

During the course of the chapter, the most important challenges for the care of the gastrointestinal surgical oncology patient will be discussed. Special attention will be paid to identifying and treating the patient at highest risk of adverse outcome. A short overview of the different tumors of the gastrointestinal tract will be provided based on tumor location, as each of these types of cancer are defined by specific characteristics. Furthermore, the most important perioperative considerations are discussed, as well as the most common complications and their management.

1.2. Types of cancer

1.2.1. Esophageal cancer

Esophageal cancer is the eighth most prevalent cancer and the sixth most frequent cause of cancer-related death worldwide. Global incidence is threefold higher in men as compared to women. With a mortality:incidence ratio of 0.88 esophageal cancer has a poor prognosis, which resulted in 400,000 deaths in 2012 [1]. Over 95% of esophageal cancers consist of squamous cell (SCC) and adenocarcinomas. Incidence of SCC is especially high in Iran and Asia (the so-called esophageal cancer belt) [3]. In Western countries, incidence of adenocarcinomas has increased substantially over the past decades, of which the most frequently affected sites are the esophagogastric junction (ECJ) and the gastric cardia [17–20]. Alcohol consumption and smoking are the main risk factors in the etiology of esophageal cancer [21–24]. Others are Barrett's esophagus, gastroesophageal reflux disease, poor diet and high body mass index [24]. Currently, radical surgical resection is considered the standard treatment for resectable esophageal carcinoma (T1-3N0-3M0) [25, 26]. Proximal and mid-esophageal tumors are approached transthoracically, distal tumors are resected through either transthoracic or transhiatal approach. Neoadjuvant chemoradiation has shown to improve local control and survival and is commonly performed [27–30]. In case of unresectable carcinomas or contraindications for surgery, chemoradiation can be performed depending on the patient's condition [31–33].

1.2.2. Gastric cancer

Gastric cancer is the fifth most prevalent cancer and the third most common cause of cancer related death worldwide. About half of all cases occur in eastern Asia [1]. There are two types of gastric adenocarcinoma: the intestinal and the diffuse type. Both can be induced by *Helicobacter pylori* infection, the primary cause of gastric cancer [34]. Gastric ulcers, adenomatous polyps and intestinal metaplasia are known precursor lesions in the intestinal type gastric cancer, while no clear precursor lesions can be indicated for the diffuse type [35]. Smoking and alcohol consumption are important risk factors, as well as dietary factors such as high salt and low vegetable intake [36, 37].

In Western countries, gastric cancer is often diagnosed at an advanced stage [38, 39]. Proximal tumors are known to be more aggressive and to have a worse prognosis compared to distal gastric cancers [40]. Curative treatment is not possible in case of distant metastasis [41], leaving only 50% of patients eligible for curative surgery. Partial or total gastrectomy is performed depending on tumor location, clinical stage, and histological type. The extent of lymphadenectomy remains a topic of debate [42, 43]. Tumors of the esophagocardial junction (ECJ) and cardia are treated, like esophageal cancers, with neoadjuvant chemoradiation. To date, there is no clear consensus in literature regarding (neo-)adjuvant therapy for noncardia gastric cancers. It has been shown, however, that perioperative chemotherapy significantly improves survival [44, 45].

1.2.3. Cancer in the liver

Most of the malignant lesions that are diagnosed in the liver are metastases from primary tumors that are located in other organs. The majority of those metastases are of colonic or rectal origin, so-called colorectal liver metastasis (CRLM). The liver is the first organ in which colorectal tumors metastasize due to the venous drainage of the gastrointestinal tract via the portal vein. Radical surgical resection is the established curative treatment for CRLM.

Partial liver resections can be performed through anatomic or nonanatomic approach, depending on tumor localization and its relation to the portal vein, hepatic vein, and hepatic artery. Important considerations for performing liver surgery for CRLM are to ensure sufficient residual liver volume after resection and to plan a radical resection. Tumor size, the number of metastases, the patient's age, narrow resection margin, extrahepatic disease, synchronicity, and primary tumor stage can all be taken into consideration but are no absolute contraindications for performing a partial liver resection for CRLM. In case, a radical surgical resection cannot be performed, radiofrequent and microwave ablation techniques and stereotactic radiotherapy can be considered as alternative treatment.

In the case of CRLM, the majority of the patients receive (neo-)adjuvant chemotherapy because of the presence of metastatic disease. Chemotherapy can be used for down staging of the tumors and to increase resectability. Because of its negative effects on the liver parenchyma, a larger residual liver volume must be ensured if chemotherapy was administered preoperatively.

Primary liver cancer occurs in the liver as well, usually as hepatocellular carcinoma (HCC). HCC has a mortality:incidence ratio of 0.95 liver cancer is the second most frequent cause of cancer death in the world, resulting in approximately 745,000 deaths in 2012 [1]. It is the sixth most prevalent cancer worldwide and incidence rates are about two- to threefold higher in men compared to women [1, 46]. Chronic liver disease (i.e., chronic hepatitis B or C infection, hereditary hemochromatosis, nonalcoholic fatty liver disease) and cirrhosis are associated with increased risk of hepatocellular carcinoma (HCC) [46–48]. Echographic surveillance in patients at increased risk can detect HCC at an earlier stage [49]. Depending on performance status, Child-Pugh classification and clinical stage, a partial liver resection or liver transplantation may be indicated [48]. Up to 80% of liver volume can be resected, provided the quality of the residual volume is high enough for regeneration and to avoid liver failure. In short, postoperative morbidity and mortality rates are only acceptable in patients with Child Pugh A and without portal hypertension. Therefore, due to liver dysfunction, most patients are ineligible for surgical treatment. Treatment options for unresectable HCC include radiofrequent ablation (RFA), percutaneous ethanol injection (PEI), transcatheter chemo-embolization (TACE), stereotactic radiotherapy, and systemic chemotherapy [50–55].

1.2.4. Pancreatic cancer

Despite diagnostic and therapeutic advances, pancreatic cancer has a very poor prognosis. It is the twelfth most prevalent cancer worldwide yet the seventh most frequent cause of cancer-related death (M:I ratio 0.98) [1]. The majority of cases occur in western countries (possibly due to underdiagnosis in less developed regions) [1]. Smoking is a main risk factor associated with increased risk of pancreatic cancer [56, 57], as well as chronic pancreatitis [58, 59], high body mass index [60, 61], and having a first-degree relative with pancreatic cancer [62–64]. The majority of tumors are ductal adenocarcinomas and over 95% arises from the exocrine elements of the pancreas. Surgical resection is considered the only potentially curative treatment, however only about 15–20% of patients are eligible for a pancreaticoduodenectomy (Whipple) [65]. Prognosis is poor even in those patients; 5-year survival is about 10% in case of node-positive and about 25–30% in node-negative disease [66–68]. Tumor characteristics are the only significant prognostic factor influencing survival after surgery [69]. Adjuvant chemotherapy has proven to improve disease free survival [70–72]. Neo-adjuvant chemoradiation, as this may improve resectability of the tumor, decreases recurrence rates [73–76]. In a palliative setting, chemotherapy and biliodigestive bypass surgery can be useful [77–81].

1.2.5. Cancers of the biliary tract

Cancers of the gallbladder and of the bile duct are less common, however, highly fatal as they are often diagnosed at an advanced stage. Gallbladder carcinoma accounts for around 1.3% of cancer incidence worldwide and is one of the few malignancies that is more common in females than in males [1, 82, 83]. Statistics on cholangiocarcinoma are less accurate as intrahepatic cholangiocarcinomas are often included in the primary liver cancers. Gallstone disease, gallbladder polyps, congenital biliary cysts, anomalous pancreaticobiliary junction, and chronic cholecystitis are predisposing factors for developing gallbladder cancer. Risk factors for cholangiocarcinoma include primary sclerosing cholangitis, choledochal cysts, chronic hepatolithiasis (recurrent pyogenic cholangitis), and chronic liver disease.

Resectability is dependent on the degree of infiltration into the proximal bileducts and liver tissue, the absence of distant metastasis and involvement of the hepatic artery and/or portal vein and the expected residual liver tissue volume [84, 85]. To ensure radical (R0) resection of these aggressive tumors, extensive liver resection and resection of other neighboring organs is sometimes necessary [86–88]. The radicality of the resection is the most important prognostic factor [89, 90]. The adequate surgical approach is selected based on tumor location and extent of tumor ingrowth. A Whipple procedure (pancreaticoduodenectomy) may be indicated in case of a distal cholangiocarcinoma. In the preoperative setting, biliary drainage and/or embolization of the portal vein may be indicated [91–94]. The role of (neo-)adjuvant chemo- and radiotherapy remains controversial and is not part of standard treatment [88, 95–97].

1.2.6. Colorectal cancer

Colorectal cancer (CRC) is the second most prevalent cancer in women, and the third most prevalent in men worldwide. The majority of cases occur in the Western world, although in recent years an increase of CRC incidence has been observed in developing countries as well, which is likely to be a consequence of the adoption of Western lifestyle and diet. CRC resulted in 694,000 deaths in 2012, which makes it the fourth most frequent cause of cancer death [1]. In developed countries, the incidence and mortality have decreased over the past decades, which is largely attributable to the implementation of better screening tools and national screening programs [98–100].

Age, adenomatous polyps, genetic factors (FAP, HNPCC), inflammatory bowel disease, history of abdominal radiotherapy, and lifestyle are the main factors associated with increased risk of colorectal cancer [101–106]. The vast majority of colorectal cancers are adenocarcinomas. All tumors originate from adenomas or flat dysplasia. Tumors of the right colon are more polypoid shaped as opposed to the annular tumors in the left colon. The prognosis for both tumor locations is, however, similar [107]. Radical resection remains the cornerstone of curative treatment. The surgical approach of choice depends on tumor location and size (i.e., right/left hemicolectomy, low anterior resection, total mesorectal excision, or abdominoperioneal resection). In case of locally advanced (T4) tumors, en-bloc multivisceral resection is advised [108, 109]. Local recurrence is more common in rectal cancer due to difficulty in obtaining adequate resection margins. In rectal cancer, neoadjuvant radiotherapy or chemoradiation may be indicated depending on disease stage. Neoadjuvant chemoradiation is also usually considered in case of locally advanced colon cancer [108]. Adjuvant chemotherapy has only proven to be beneficial for lymph node positive colon cancer.

2. Current challenges in gastrointestinal, hepatobiliary, and pancreatic surgical oncology

2.1. Frail elderly

With the aging of the population, patients undergoing surgery for gastrointestinal and hepatobiliary and pancreatic cancers are also becoming older: one of every three cancers is diagnosed in patients aged 65 years or older. A more worrying fact, however, is that the majority of cancer-related deaths occur in this group of patients [110]. Older patients are at increased risk for perioperative complications [111], which may lead to prolonged hospital stay, decreased quality of life and independency, increased disability and health-care costs, and increased mortality [112]. Nevertheless, carefully selected patients seem to benefit from surgery in the long-term [113]. Therefore, preoperative risk assessment, and multimodal perioperative care for elderly patients remain of paramount importance in the light of changing patient demographics [114]. Various risk classification systems, such as the American Society for Anesthesiologists (ASA) classification, Charlson Comorbidity Index, and the Eastern Cooperative Oncology Group (ECOG) performance status, have been developed to categorize patients' preoperative condition [115–117]. However, many of these classifications are inaccurate; they are subjective or focus on a single organ system [118]. The ASA classification for instance, shows large intraobserver variability [116, 119], and lacks specificity for cancer patients, who are known to have an altered metabolism that may affect ASA-score.

Factors contributing to an impaired postoperative outcome for vulnerable (elderly) patients are frequently referred to as "frailty." Frailty has gained attention as a risk factor for adverse outcome after surgery over the past decades. Screening for and the assessment of frailty can aid risk assessment and therefore facilitate the decision making process for both patients and physicians. The concept of frailty was defined as a biologic syndrome, characterized by a decreased reserve and resistance to stressors [12, 109]. It incorporates a number of areas of functioning, including weight loss, muscle weakness (e.g., grip strength), slowness, low activity, and increased disability [12]. Increased 6-month mortality was observed in frail individuals in a study of patients who underwent major surgery (i.e., procedures that required standard ICU admission) [120]. Geriatric markers for frailty (e.g., cognitive function, poor nutritional status, falls, depressed mood, and anemia) were predictive for adverse outcome in this study [120]. Furthermore, increased complication rate and length of stay were observed in frail patients who underwent elective surgery [121]. Finally, frailty was shown to be associated with increased surgical complications, postoperative mortality, health care costs, and length of stay [118, 120, 122].

2.2. Sarcopenia and cachexia

A modifiable, hallmark sign of frailty is sarcopenia, a geriatric term for the involuntary loss of skeletal muscle mass and density [123–125]. The prevalence of sarcopenia increases with age; from 9% at 45 years to 64% at 85 years in healthy ambulatory individuals [126]. This condition is characterized by a loss of skeletal muscle mass and strength [127], leading to physical impairment and disability in geriatric populations [128, 129]. Multiple studies have shown an association between the presence of sarcopenia and adverse outcome after surgery. For instance, following surgery for colorectal liver metastases, sarcopenia negatively affected short-term outcome with increased morbidity and mortality rates In a study published in 2011 [130]. Sarcopenia also negatively influenced long-term outcome in patients who underwent surgery for pancreatic adenocarcinoma (i.e., 3-year survival), as well as for patients undergoing surgery for colorectal liver metastases (i.e., 5-year disease free and overall survival) [131, 132]. Similar studies found an unusually high prevalence of sarcopenia (57.7% of 180 patients) in Western gastric cancer patients [133]. However, this study did not find any association with adverse outcomes in patients with sarcopenia. Another recent study in Asian gastric cancer patients described a much lower prevalence of sarcopenia (12.5% of 255 patients). This study combined CT-scan measurements with hand-grip strength and get-up-and-go tests to define sarcopenia. In this study, sarcopenia was found to be an independent risk factor for postoperative complications [134]. Besides sarcopenia, older cancer patients may also suffer from cancer induced cachexia, a clinical condition leading to skeletal muscle loss with or without the loss of adipose tissue due to anorexia (resulting from e.g. metabolic changes) and malnutrition (resulting from e.g. (chemotherapy induced) nausea and loss of appetite) [135, 136]. It is estimated that cachexia is the cause of up to 30% of cancer related deaths [137, 138]. Sarcopenia and cachexia are therefore separate but overlapping entities, with different pathways that both lead to skeletal muscle wasting [139]. The assessment of sarcopenia will be elucidated further in the third paragraph.

2.3. Body composition and chemotherapy

Although surgery remains the cornerstone of curative cancer treatment in all gastrointestinal and hepatopancreatobiliary malignancies, a substantial part of patients is treated with chemotherapy [29, 140]. This could be either in a neoadjuvant setting to reduce the tumor load, as well as in an adjuvant or palliative setting in patients with locally advanced/metastasized disease or recurrence, respectively.

A recent report described that skeletal muscle loss during neoadjuvant chemotherapy is associated with poor short-term outcome in esophageal cancer patients [141]. Two other studies did not find an association with overall (long-term) survival [142, 143]. In a study among breast cancer patients who received neoadjuvant therapy, sarcopenic patients were more likely to have a complete pathologic response compared to nonsarcopenic patients [144]. Substantial loss of body weight, adipose tissue and skeletal muscle mass have been reported among pancreatic cancer patients who received neoadjuvant radiochemotherapy within phase I and II clinical trials. [145, 146]. Although the resection rate could not be predicted by body composition parameters (i.e., weight loss, overweight/obesity (pre-/posttreatment), sarcopenia with or without overweight/obesity), the extent of skeletal muscle and visceral adipose tissue loss was negatively associated with disease-free survival and overall- and progression-free survival, respectively [145]. Finally, an increasing number of studies show that low skeletal muscle mass is an independent determinant of chemotherapy toxicity in different patient populations treated with various chemotherapeutics [147–153]. Chemotherapy toxicity frequently leads to dose limitation or abortion of therapy. Consequently, this may lead to less effective cancer treatment and impaired (disease-free) survival. Therefore, it is suggested that it would be better to base dose normalization on skeletal muscle mass rather than body surface area (BSA), as is commonly performed [147].

3. Identifying the patient with high perioperative risk

3.1. Preoperative assessment

Risk assessment in order to identify patients at risk for postoperative adverse events is a complex effort. It is made even more difficult by the great variety of primary diseases as well as comorbidities in surgical oncology patients.

Classically, preoperative risk assessment is based on a complex interaction of the clinician's view of the general status of the patient and The consideration of factors such as age, comorbidities and ASA classification. This can be a subjective process and its interpretation can vary greatly between clinicians. Even the assessment of the ASA classification seems to be a relatively subjective process [154]. Consultation of an experienced anesthesiologist is often advised for patients with a compromised physical status (e.g., ASA 3–4) or who are scheduled to undergo major surgical interventions that can cause physiological derangements.

3.2. Risk factors for adverse outcome

Gastrointestinal surgical oncology patients are often elderly patients. The elderly are at an increased risk for adverse events and mortality [155, 156]. A patient's ability to cope with surgical stressors is determined by a multitude of factors, of which physiological reserves are the most important. In recent years, improvements have been made to identify more objective risk factors for adverse outcome after surgery. These include comorbidity classifications, geriatric frailty assessment, sarcopenia, and malnutrition assessment.

3.3. Comorbidities

Almost all patients who undergo major gastrointestinal surgery have some degree of comorbidity. In order to classify these comorbidities and to determine a risk stratification for mortality, the Charlson Comorbidity Index (CCI) was introduced [115]. This index was also used for prediction of mortality risk after complex gastrointestinal surgery in a later study [157]. In Asian elderly patients (octo- and nonagenarians) undergoing surgery for gastric cancer, a CCI ≥ 5 was associated with a higher postoperative mortality rate [158]. In another study in elderly Italian patients who underwent curative surgery for gastric cancer, the presence of comorbidity and not age was the only independent risk factor for mortality [130].

3.4. Frailty

Assessment of frailty as depicted above can be diverse and often incorporates different measurement modalities. These include questionnaires on self-reported health and disability, handgrip strength measurements, timed get-up-and-go tests and sometimes blood tests (hemoglobin, albumin). These measurements make frailty assessment difficult in an outpatient setting. Therefore, fast and easy to perform screening questionnaires have been developed over the recent years. Examples include PRISMA-7, Fried's Frailty criteria, Hopkins Frailty score and Groningen Frailty Indicator (GFI) [159]. Questionnaires such as the GFI encompass multiple aspects of frailty, i.e., mobility, physical fitness, vision, hearing, nourishment (i.e., unintended weight loss), morbidity (i.e., polypharmacy), and psychosocial status [14]. Despite the comprehensive nature of these questionnaires, the percentage of patients who are identified as frail vary strongly between different risk assessment tools (11.6–36.4%) [159]. However, these questionnaires have proved to be very useful to identify patients who are at risk for the development of postoperative adverse events. In gastric cancer patients, a GFI ≥3 was associated with postoperative mortality and morbidity (severe complications) [160]. Frail patients had an in-hospital mortality of 23.3% compared to 5.2% for nonfrail patients. Scores higher than 7 on the Edmonton Frail scale were associated with increased complications after non-cardiac surgery (OR 5.02, 95% CI 1.55–16.25) [121]. In another study, Fried's Frailty criteria were associated with increased complications after major, oncological and urological surgeries [118]. Geriatric assessment using several questionnaires was used in a study and showed that frailty is an independent risk factor for impaired 1-year and 5-year survival after colorectal cancer surgery [161].

In conclusion, frailty screening and assessment with referral to a geriatric specialist should be included in preoperative work-up and shared decision making in elderly patients scheduled to undergo gastrointestinal surgery for cancer.

3.5. Sarcopenia

A decline in muscle mass, or sarcopenia, is a phenomenon within the process of human aging but is also part of the cachexia syndrome [127, 162]. Sarcopenia is a complex syndrome and multiple factors have been identified that contribute to its development [163]. Inadequate nutrition (low protein intake and impaired metabolism) and inactivity are important contributing elements, as well as age-related and possibly endocrine factors [127].

The assessment of sarcopenia is performed by measuring muscle surface areas on abdominal CT-scans. At a designated level (e.g., transverse processes of lumbar spine L3), total psoas cross-sectional area or total muscle surface area are measured and corrected for patient height, resulting in an L3-index (see **Figure 2**). These measurements can be performed in a semiautomated fashion by the use of image analysis software. Sex and body mass index (BMI) specific cutoffs are available to define sarcopenia. For instance: for men 43 cm^2/m^2 (BMI < 25.0 kg/m^2) and 53 cm^2/m^2 (BMI ≥ 25.0 kg/m^2), in women L3-index lower than 41 cm^2/m^2 [164].

Sarcopenia, as measured by low muscle mass CT-scans, is used in a multitude of studies and has been shown to be associated with adverse outcome. However, in 2010, the European Working Group on Sarcopenia in Older People (EWGSOP) defined sarcopenia as a low muscle mass in combination with either low muscle strength or low physical activity [127]. The EWGSOP defines low muscle mass as only symptom as presarcopenia.

3.6. Malnutrition

An imbalance in energy expenditure and nutritional intake is the fundamental physiological derangement that causes cancer-induced weight loss. Tumor-related factors that contribute to weight loss include early satiety, obstruction complaints, but also tumor induced metabolic changes [162]. Especially, upper GI cancer patients are at risk for malnutrition, for example, in 31-43% of gastric cancer patients there can be a weight loss of >10% in the last 6 months. [165]. Malnutrition is a well-known risk factor for adverse outcomes after upper GI surgery, including interventions for esophageal, gastric cancer, liver and pancreatic cancer [162, 166, 167].

SNAQ Short Nutritional Assessment Questionnaire	
- Did you lose weight unintentionally? More than 6 kg in the last 6 month More than 3kg in the last month	 ••• ••
- Did you experience a decreased appetite over the last months?	•
- Did you use supplemental drinks or tube feeding over the last month?	•
• No intervention •• Moderately malnourished; nutritional intervention ••• Severely malnourished; nutritional intervention and treatment dietician	

MUST Malnutrition Universal Screening Tool	
Have you/the patient lost weight recently without trying? No Unsure Yes, How much (kg)? 1-5 6-10 11-15 > 15 Unsure	 0 2 1 2 3 4 2
Have you/the patient been eating poorly because of a decreased appetite? No Yes	 0 1
Do you feel you look frail or under your most comfortable weight? No Yes	 0 1

Figure 1. Short Nutritional Assessment Questionnaire (SNAQ) and Malnutrition Universal Screening Tool (MUST). Partly adapted from Kruizenga et al. [15] and Rahman et al. [16].

Screening for malnutrition is therefore an important aspect of the preoperative risk assessment of upper GI cancer patients. Several questionnaires have been developed to screen for malnutrition, which include: NRS-2002 (nutritional risk screening), MUST (Malnutrition Universal Screening Tool), SNAQ (Short Nutritional Assessment Questionnaire) [15, 160, 168] (**Figure 1**).

These tools provide an easy and low-cost method for nutritional risk stratification and provide an indication as to when preoperative nutritional interventions are indicated. Patients at risk for malnutrition should be referred to a dietician for nutritional analysis and supplementation if needed, in order to optimize preoperative status.

3.7. Patient selection

Upper GI cancer patients are scheduled to undergo major surgery if they are considered "fit for surgery." Proper preoperative evaluation can identify avoidable perioperative risks. As upper GI cancer surgery is often performed in elderly patients, chronic comorbidities are frequently present.

Basic preoperative assessment, including clinical history taking and physical examination, should aim at identifying chronic comorbidities. Preoperative evaluation should uncover any chronic comorbidities, particularly cardiovascular and pulmonary disease [169]. Advice from other departments should be obtained, e.g., adjustment of pulmonary medications and corticosteroid supplementation in patients with pulmonary disease. This helps minimizing avoidable perioperative cardiopulmonary complications.

Another important risk factor for adverse outcome is the presence of diabetes mellitus. This should therefore be optimally controlled pre- and perioperatively. If necessary, referral to a specialist is recommended.

Referral to a geriatric specialist can be very helpful in the preoperative setting, especially for frail elderly. Advice can be obtained in the perioperative stage on prevention of delirium, and of physical and cognitive decline.

Exercise tolerance is also an important aspect to judge physiological reserves. It is most often determined by the patient's cardiopulmonary limitations. Metabolic equivalents of a task (MET) can be helpful with assessing exercise tolerance. Patients who are able to perform four MET's or greater are regarded to have a low risk for perioperative morbidity [169]. Climbing a flight of stairs roughly equates to four MET's; when patients are able to do so, they are considered to be fit for elective surgery.

When patients are adequately evaluated, risks can be communicated between treating physicians, patients and family members. If the patient is deemed fit for surgery, these preoperative consultations help provide an optimal perioperative environment for patients and minimize the risk of preventable complications.

4. Standardized care by the use of clinical pathways

An increasing number of surgical procedures are performed each year for abdominal malignant diseases. The indications for surgery are expanding and the surgical techniques are becoming more sophisticated. However, surgical morbidity remains high, especially after major abdominal surgery such as gastric, esophageal, liver, pancreatic or colorectal surgery. There is an increasing need for protocoled care and new care pathways for surgery to reduce surgical impact and perioperative morbidity [170].

Since the last decade of the twentieth century, fast-track or enhanced recovery care protocols for surgical care gained popularity. These clinical pathways are aimed at reducing surgical morbidity by reducing the perioperative physiological and psychological stress and enhancing patients' recovery (see **Figure 2**) [171, 172]. The physiological changes a patient must endure during and after surgery are influenced by many different factors. Therefore, enhanced recovery pathways are aimed at a multimodal approach in which the surgeon, anesthesiologist, nurse, nutritionist, and physiotherapist all contribute in improving the patient's recovery [173–175].

As mentioned before, the surgical stress is influenced by many factors, such as the surgical procedure itself, intraoperative hypothermia, low glucose levels due to perioperative fasting, intraoperative anesthetics, pain, and being bedridden. These stressors are specific targets for enhanced recovery pathways. The key elements in enhanced recovery pathways are minimized preoperative fasting, limited use of incisions, catheters, and drains, early resumption of oral diet, early mobilization after surgery and optimal pain control using patient controlled (epidural) analgesia [170, 173, 174, 176–178].

These elements relieve patients of previously described stressors that are the cause of postoperative morbidity and delayed recovery. The result of enhanced recovery pathways can be seen in a reduction of postoperative complications and subsequently a shortening of median hospital stay [179–181].

Preoperative factors
Preadmission counseling
Fluid and carbohydrate loading
No prolonged fasting
No/selective bowel preparation
Antibiotic prophylaxis
Thrombopropylaxis
No premedication

Intraoperative factors
Short-acting anesthetic agents
No drains
Avoidance of salt and water overload
Maintenance of normothermia

Enhanced Care

Postoperative factors
Mid-thoracic epidural anesthesia/analgesia
No nasogastric tubes
Prevention of nausea and vomiting
Early removal of catheter
Early oral nutrition
Non-opioid oral analgesia/NSAIDs
Early mobilization
Stimulation of gut motility
Audit of compliance and outcomes

Figure 2. Important elements of enhanced care protocols for perioperative care.

4.1. Upper GI surgery

4.1.1. Standardized postoperative care

A number of general enhanced recovery pathways developed for colorectal cancer are also applicable to esophageogastric surgery patients. Aspects that will be discussed in this section are preoperative nutrition, timing of postoperative oral intake, use of nasogastric and decompression catheters, early mobilization, and urinary catheter use.

As stated before, malnutrition is associated with adverse outcome in esophagogastric surgery [182, 183]. Although evidence for preoperative feeding interventions is limited [184], it is still recommended to screen for and treat malnutrition in gastroesophageal cancer patients by optimization of nutritional intake with oral feeding supplements [178, 185]. Dietary interventions have not shown to be beneficial in patients who do not suffer from malnutrition [186].

Nasogastric decompression recommendations during the postoperative phase are different after gastric and esophageal surgery. Evidence against nasogastric decompression after gastrectomy is strong, as several meta-analyses show deleterious effects of routine nasogastric tube placement [187, 188]. Furthermore, its routine use does not reduce surgical morbidity. Additionally, patients without decompression have fewer pulmonary complications, earlier passage of flatus, earlier resumption of oral intake, and a shorter length of stay [188].

In patients undergoing esophagectomy, in contrast to gastrectomy patients, gastric conduit decompression is recommended. The aim of the nasogastric tube is to prevent gastric stasis, pain, vomiting, and aspiration. On the other hand, nasogastric tubes are associated with increased epistaxis, dislodgement of the catheter, and pulmonary infections [189]. One RCT that studied the effect of nasogastric tube decompression, however, found a reduction in pulmonary complications [190]. All in all, gastric conduit decompression via nasogastric tube is recommended [185].

Timing of resumption of oral diet is challenging after gastrectomy and esophagectomy with important differences between the two. After gastrectomy, there is evidence to support early resumption of liquid intake (the first day following surgery) and to further increase this according to tolerance, starting with light food on day two [178]. Conversely, there are no studies that report adverse outcome after early and patient controlled introduction of oral diet in gastrectomy patients [178].

Resumption of oral intake after esophagectomy is somewhat unclear and traditionally conservative. There are some studies that have investigated early oral intake after gastric and gastroesophageal resection [191, 192]. After total gastrectomy ($n = 77$) and esophagectomy ($n = 2$), earlier discharge was seen in the enteral feeding group [192]. However, no esophagectomy-specific studies have been published on this subject, which makes it difficult to give evidence-based recommendations.

After esophagogastric surgery, nutritional support is indicated if 60% of desired oral intake is not achieved by the end of the first week, as is suggested by a large review [162]. High-energy oral sip feeds is the preferred method, but enteral tube feeding can be used when this is not possible.

Strong evidence exists that bed rest is associated with several adverse outcomes. For example, even in healthy individuals, bed rest has been shown to decrease maximal oxygen uptake (VO2 max) [193]. Despite this, very few specific postoperative protocols have been developed with good evidence-based support [194]. Nonetheless, early postoperative mobilization from day one, which can be supported by written day-to-day patient instructions, is regarded as good practice [178, 185]. Adequate analgesia is a requirement for effective early mobilization.

Urinary catheters are often used for patients monitoring, especially in the early postoperative stage. However, there are some notable disadvantages for the use of catheters, including restricted patient mobility and an increased risk of urinary tract infection. Furthermore, they have shown to be a predictor for longer length of stay [195]. Transurethral catheters can and should be removed on day one or two postoperatively if the presence of the catheter is not required for monitoring [178].

In conclusion, many aspects of enhanced recovery pathways can be implemented in upper GI surgery. However, there are some points specific to upper GI that require special attention. These include the use of nasogastric tubes, early mobilization, timing of resumption of oral diet, and use of urinary catheters. These points are generally not well studied but recommendations for daily practice can be made using the available evidence as outlined above.

4.2. Colorectal surgery

4.2.1. Colorectal surgery

Colorectal carcinoma (CRC) is the fourth most common cancer worldwide for both males and females. Surgery remains an important aspect of curative treatment of CRC, and also the patient in the palliative setting is frequently operated on due to the obstructive nature of the disease. Perioperative care for patients undergoing colorectal surgery has improved significantly over the past decades, mainly due to the introduction of enhanced recovery pathways and the implementation of less invasive surgical techniques. It has been shown that these programs have a positive influence on the duration of the hospital admission and overall complication rate [196].

The recommendations that are supported by grade A evidence will be further elucidated in this section. Furthermore, recommendations that require further high quality research will be mentioned here as well.

Preoperative preparation of the patient includes fasting protocols and mechanical bowel preparation. Recent guidelines have altered the traditional nil by mouth period (fasting from midnight) to a minimum period of two hours, based on a high-quality meta-analysis [197]. It has been shown that prolonged fasting before surgery does not increase the pH of gastric content nor does it influence the aspiration risk during and after surgery.

Mechanical bowel preparation (MBP) has been used in combination with oral antibiotic therapy since the 70's to decrease the bacterial load in the bowel lumen prior to surgery. However, from the many studies have been conducted since, no convincing evidence arose regarding the beneficial effects of MBP alone, which in part explains why MBP has been abandoned in many institutions. In fact, several articles described possible harmful effects associated with mechanically cleansing the bowel, such as prolonged postoperative ileus and spillage of bowel content into the abdominal cavity [198]. However, none of these studies included an arm where a combination of MBP and oral antibiotics was compared to MBP and oral antibiotics alone. Furthermore, several studies have shown a reduced length of stay and lower risk of surgical site infection when patients were subjected to both oral and mechanical bowel preparation [199, 200].

Another important change that has been observed in daily practice is the intravenous administration of antibiotics as opposed to oral administration, mostly because of practical reasons. A recently conducted Cochrane Review has focused on the timing, type and administration route of antibiotic prophylaxis and, but concluded that robust evidence on this is still lacking [201]. It seems that a combination of oral and intravenous prophylaxis is most effective in decreasing the risk of surgical site infection, as are antibiotics that cover both aerobic and anaerobic bacteria [201]. For intravenous antibiotics, it is generally accepted that the optimal timing of administration is 30–60 min before surgery [202]. No recommendations can be made for timing of oral antibiotics based on the available literature.

An important way of reducing the surgical stress is the use of epidural analgesia. It reduces the use of opioids during the postoperative phase, which in turn provides rapid awakening, early intake and mobilization, and therefore improves gastrointestinal motility [203]. Besides the adverse effects on postoperative ileus, important side effects of opioids on the respiratory function and central nervous system have been described [204]. There is an important lack of level A evidence against the use of NSAIDs during the postoperative phase. However, retrospective data and animal studies have shown an increased risk for anastomotic leakage with the use of NSAIDs [205–207]. It is therefore recommended to refrain from the prescription of NSAIDs following colorectal surgery.

4.3. HPB surgery

In some centers worldwide that perform hepatopancreatobiliary surgery, similar enhanced recovery pathways have been implemented as to those that have been described in the previous sections for gastroesophageal and colorectal surgery. Naturally, there are similarities between the pathways for gastrointestinal surgery and HPB surgery such as early resumption of oral intake, early mobilization, the use of laxatives postoperatively and the use of epidural analgesia [176, 208, 209]. There are, however, a number of important specific considerations for enhanced care pathways in the field of liver and pancreatic surgery that will be addressed in this section.

4.3.1. Liver surgery

Laparoscopic surgery is being practiced increasingly more in the field of abdominal surgery in general and has become the gold standard for many procedures such as the cholecystectomy. Minimal invasive keyhole surgery decreases postoperative morbidity and facilitates faster recovery after surgery. Minimizing incisions is one of the elements of many enhanced care pathways for that reason. Due to surgical technical challenges, the laparoscopic approach for liver surgery was introduced later than for gastrointestinal surgery. In the early period of laparoscopic liver surgery, only minor liver resections were performed, such as the left lateral sectionectomy [210]. Today, the number of laparoscopic liver surgery procedures is growing both for minor and major liver resections, yielding promising results [211, 212].

Traditionally, the placement of prophylactic intra-abdominal drains after liver surgery is a strategy that has been used for the early detection of postresectional hemorrhage and bile leakage. Intra-abdominal drains, however, have negative effects as well; they can cause ascending intra-abdominal infections and can be uncomfortable for the patient, thereby delaying postoperative recovery. In this day and age, with improved abilities to perform CT- or ultrasound-guided drainage of intra-abdominal fluid collections, abdominal drains have become obsolete for uncomplicated partial liver resection when regarding the number of postoperative complications and reinterventions [213]. In some cases, the use of a prophylactic drain can be advocated, for example, when surgery with vascular or biliary reconstruction is performed or when, in the case of central liver resection, the risk of a postoperative biloma or hemorrhage increases [214, 215].

4.3.2. Pancreatic surgery

Pancreatic adenocarcinomas are notorious for causing severe weight loss in patients, and, as mentioned before, cachexia is an important challenge in this patient group. Therefore, an optimal preoperative nutritional status is a key element in the enhanced recovery pathways for pancreatic surgery. Fortunately, the majority of the patients that undergo a pancreatic resection are not malnourished and have minor to intermediate weight loss. This group does not need additional nutritional support. However, patients that do suffer from severe weight loss and are in a state of malnourishment are in need of receiving additional nutrition. This can be administered either by oral supplements or by enteral tube feeding if necessary [176, 216].

Cholestasis is one of the side effects of pancreatic carcinoma. This occurs when the common bile duct is obstructed by the tumor mass. Preoperative biliary drainage of the common bile duct should be considered in severe jaundiced patients. Preoperative biliary drainage can be performed by the placement of a stent in the common bile duct via endoscopic retrograde cholangiopancreatography (ERCP). When the common bile duct is inaccessible via ERCP due to impassable obstruction in the bile duct or duodenum, biliary drainage can be performed via percutaneous transhepatic cholangiography (PTHC). A serum bilirubin concentration >250 μmol/l is associated with an increased risk of postoperative morbidity. Patients with a higher serum concentration of bilirubin should therefore receive preoperative biliary drainage [176, 217].

In most enhanced recovery protocols, the routine use of prophylactic abdominal drains after surgery is discouraged because of drain-related morbidity. There has been a recent debate on the routine use of prophylactic abdominal drains after pancreaticoduodenectomy (PD). After a PD, an abdominal drain is normally placed for early detection of anastomotic leakage or hemorrhage. Leakages of the pancreaticojejunostomy or the hepaticojejunostomy can have detrimental effects and are potentially lethal. However, drain-related complications have also been reported, and earlier studies with small patient groups showed promising results regarding postoperative complications in patients that were treated without a prophylactic abdominal drain [218]. In addition, early drain removal was shown to be beneficial for postoperative morbidity [219]. In a recent RCT, the abandonment of prophylactic drain use had a detrimental effect on postoperative mortality. Therefore, prophylactic drain use is still advised for safe postoperative care after PD in all patients [220, 221]. In the coming years, new evidence will have to show if the use of prophylactic abdominal drains can be abandoned in low-risk patients undergoing a PD.

4.4. ICU care

4.4.1. Handover

The transfer from the operating theatre to the intensive care unit is the first step in standardized postoperative care, and should therefore be considered a crucial one. Agarwal et al. report a substantial improvement in quality of the handover when using a standardized and structured method of communication in pediatric patients who underwent cardiac surgery. They compared the knowledge of medical providers regarding patient information following the handover by means of a questionnaire. The knowledge of the clinical team members after the structured handover was 92% compared to 69% in case of the verbal handover. Furthermore, the outcome differences between these two groups were assessed. In the verbal handover group, 5.4% were in need of cardiopulmonary resuscitation compared to 2.6% in case of the structured handover ($p = 0.043$). The same was true for the need of mediastinal re-exploration: 9% versus 5.5% respectively ($p = 0.043$). Metabolic acidosis occurred in 6.7% of cases of verbal handover versus 2.6% structured handover ($p = 0.004$) and successful early extubation could be conducted in 43.2% and 50% respectively ($p = 0.04$). It could therefore be concluded that a structured handover should be a part of the standardized postoperative care.

4.4.2. Extubation

Early extubation is known to be a predictive factor for early discharge. Cheng et al. already stated that early extubation led to a decrease of 25% of the total costs of CABG surgery. This cost reduction is a result of early discharge of the ICU and, consequently, from the hospital itself. Consequences for the patients are not described in this article but can be imagined. In cases of intubation, patients are often sedated and immobile. Immobilization induces a significant decrease in muscle mass and strength. As stated before, the loss of muscle mass strongly hampers recovery in oncological surgery.

4.4.3. Mobilization

Mobilization is a crucial part of enhanced recovery programs that has been explained earlier in this chapter. In case of ICU admittance, the patient usually receives cardiovascular support by means of vasopressin or respiratory support by mechanic ventilation and oxygenation. Obviously, these conditions make mobilization rather difficult. However, Brahmbhatt et al. conducted an intervention-based study in which the intervention group ($n = 49$) was subjected to daily interruptions of sedation. Patients in the intervention group received physical and occupational therapy during the earliest days of critical illness. Outcome parameters were functional status at hospital discharge, duration of delirium and ventilator-free days during the first 28 days. In 29 patients (59%) of the intervention group independent functional status was reached compared to 19 patients (35%) of the control group ($n = 55$) ($p = 0.02$). Furthermore, a shorter period of delirium (median 2 days) was observed in the intervention group compared to 4 days in the control group ($p = 0.02$), as well as a significant increase in ventilator free days: 23.5 versus 21.1 days respectively ($p = 0.05$).

http://dx.doi.org/10.5772/64775

4.4.4. Complication management

The intensive care unit uses several instruments to increase insight into risk management. The most used and internationally recognized are the Simplified Acute Physiologic Score (SAPS), Sequential Organ Failure Assessment (SOFA), ASA-score, and Acute Physiology and Chronic Health Evaluation (APACHE score).

4.4.5. SAPS score

The Simplified Acute Physiologic Score, otherwise known as SAPS, can be used to predict hospital mortality. Patients with a higher SAPS score have a higher mortality. The latest version of the SAPS score instrument is SAPS II. SAPS III has also recently been validated. Recent studies show a good discrimination by SAPS III, but a poor calibration.

4.4.6. SOFA score

The SOFA score consists of six different scores, which are organ specific. These score the respiratory, nervous, renal, and cardiovascular system, liver and coagulation. Each item can be scored between one and four, which results in a score between seven and 28.

American Society of Anesthesiologist (ASA) Physical Status

Category	Description
ASA 1	Healthy patient
ASA 2	Mild to moderate systemic disease caused by the surgical condition or by other pathological processes, and medically well controlled
ASA 3	Severe disease process which limits activity but is not incapacitating
ASA 4	Severe incapacitating disease process that is a constant threat to life
ASA 5	Moribund patient not expected to survive 24h with or without an operation

Figure 3. American Society of Anesthesiologist (ASA) categorization.

4.4.7. ASA classification score

Originally, the ASA physical status classification system was developed by the American Society of Anesthesiologists and consisted of five categories (see **Figure 3**). The system was designed to have a quick method to classify the physical fitness of patients. Later a sixth category was added.

4.4.8. APACHE score

The APACHE score was originally designed for patients in the intensive care unit. The designers were trying to develop a quantification method for the severity of disease of ICU-admitted patients.

The score is calculated by the use of different parameters: PaO_2, temperature, mean arterial pressure, arterial pH, heart rate, respiratory rate, Glasgow Coma Scale and blood analysis for sodium, potassium, creatinine, hematocrit, and white blood cell count. All of these measurements should be conducted in the first 24 hours of admission; the score should not be changed during the course of admission. The latest version is the APACHE IV, which has been constructed using a new logistical regression equation, a different set of variables and statistical modeling to improve accuracy.

5. Improving postoperative outcome

5.1. Cardiopulmonary exercise testing

With expanding indications for surgery and a population that grows increasingly older, patient selection for extensive surgery becomes more important. To assess if patients are fit for major abdominal surgery, surgeons and anesthesiologists need objective tools. Cardiopulmonary exercise testing (CPET) can be used as an objective instrument to assess the cardiopulmonary fitness of a patient in an outpatient setting.

The test originated from exercise physiology, and was later adopted by other clinical departments for the determination of physical condition. Since recent years, different surgical departments use CPET to objectively assess high-risk patients before taking the patients to the operation theatre.

Cardiopulmonary exercise testing is an objective way to assess a patient's maximal cardiorespiratory fitness. CPET is performed on a cycling ergometer or on a treadmill. During the test, ventilation gas exchange parameters are measured by breath analysis and cardiac parameters are monitored by electrocardiogram. Ventilation gas analysis is used to determine oxygen and carbon dioxide exchange. Different protocols can be used for CPET, but cycling ergometry with an incremental or 'ramped' workload is most common [222].

By gradually increasing the workload for the patient, the oxygen demand in the muscles also increases. When the oxygen demand exceeds oxygen delivery, the anaerobic threshold (AT) is passed. The AT, together with the maximal or peak oxygen uptake (VO_{2peak}),is valuable parameters which reflect the maximal cardiopulmonary capacity of a patient [222].

Several CPET-derived variables have been associated with morbidity, mortality and length of stay after major intra-abdominal surgery, in particular the AT and VO_{2peak}. Hence, CPET can be used to identify patients with decreased cardiopulmonary reserve, which are those patients who have an increased risk for morbidity and mortality after major intra-abdominal surgery [223–225].

Subsequently, patients with an increased perioperative risk based upon low CPET scores can be offered preoperative exercise therapy or so-called prehabilitation prior to surgery to improve their fitness and thereby reducing perioperative risk.

5.2. Prehabilitation/exercise interventions

Prehabilitation and exercise interventions can be applied in frail elderly to reduce the risks of perioperative morbidity and mortality. The main intention of exercise is to counter the weight loss and therefore improve muscle strength and function. This will consequently lead to improved daily functioning and better quality of life in these patients.

Even though resistance exercise is known to increase muscle strength in older patients, it seems to have little effect on the actual muscle mass itself. However, several reviews and meta-analyses found an improved physical functioning and overall quality of life in cancer patients from physical exercise [226, 227]. Furthermore, it has been shown that low or decreased physical functioning in the preoperative phase is associated with postoperative complications [228, 229].

In addition to the role of exercise, nutritional intake has an important influence on physical functioning as well. Elderly often have a poor intake, which hampers muscle development and strengthening. It has been shown that the intake of amino acids combined with physical exercise elicits the greatest anabolic response [230], and that essential amino acids in particular stimulate muscle protein synthesis [231]. Beta-hydroxy-beta-methylbutyrate (HMB) has shown to be a promising effective nutritional supplement in the increase of protein turnover [232]. When in older men and women HMB supplementation was combined with a resistance training program, an increase in lean body mass and decrease in body fat was observed, when compared to the placebo group. [233]. When older men and women were administered additional nutrition supplements with HMB, their functionality, strength, and lean body mass improved [234], as did their protein turnover [235]. Other studies have found a positive effect of whey protein on protein turnover rates when consumed within 1 hour after their exercise regimen [236].

Recently, the PACES study (Physical exercise during Adjuvant Chemotherapy Effectiveness Study), experienced beneficial effects from exercise on functionality. In this study, 230 patients with breast cancer were included and got either a home-based physical activity program (Onco-Move), a moderate to high-intensity supervised training combined with resistance and aerobic exercise (OnTrack) or usual care program. Patients with either the Onco-Move or OnTrack program showed less decline in their cardiorespiratory fitness and physical functioning. They also showed less nausea, vomiting and pain during their therapy compared to the usual care program. Both intervention groups returned to work sooner and worked more hours per week compared to the control group [237].

As noted before, multiple dimensions can be assessed when evaluating frailty. In addition to physical parameters, emotional factors and cognition should be assessed as well [238]. Indeed, psychotherapy has showed to significantly reduce fatigue in patients who were treated for cancer [239]. Furthermore, interventions with a more general approach, aiming at psychological distress, mood and physical symptoms, are effective in reducing fatigue [240].

5.3. Dietary interventions/optimized nutrition

Malnutrition is very common amongst the hospitalized population as a whole, and the prevalence increases even further for patients undergoing surgery for upper gastrointestinal or colorectal malignancies [241, 242]. It has been stated that around 50% of all patients undergoing surgery for cancer suffer from malnutrition. It is associated with adverse outcomes, including increased morbidity and mortality and decreased quality of life. Furthermore, it has been shown to be a prognostic indicator for disease specific survival in various types of cancers [243]. Interestingly, and despite the important impact malnutrition has on health care costs, the assessment of nutritional status has not yet been implemented in daily practice [244].

Several factors have been identified that predispose patients to malnutrition, including anorexia, cachexia and the early satiety sensation frequently experienced by individuals with cancer. Furthermore, metabolic alterations induced by the presence of the tumor or tumor factors can compromise nutritional status. An increased inflammatory status, which is often observed in patients suffering from a malignancy, can trigger a cascade of molecular events, including increased lipolysis and muscle proteolysis, a syndrome referred to as cancer cachexia [245]. Cachexia has been especially well described for patients with solid tumors of the pancreas and upper gastrointestinal tract and less often in patients with lower gastrointestinal cancer.

Clinicians have been aware of the importance of nutritional status for surgical outcome for over 80 years. Surprisingly, this has not yet led to the development of a generally accepted screening system for malnourished patients or patients at risk for malnourishment. Several screening tools have been proposed and validated for this purpose: the nutritional risk index (NRI), prognostic nutritional index (PNI), subjective global assessment (SGA), malnutrition universal screening tool (MUST) and short nutritional screening questionnaire (SNAQ) to name some. These tools, together with certain anthropometric measurements, such as body mass index (BMI) and serum markers of nutrition (e.g. albumin) can aid in the risk assessment and the development of a treatment plan. Significant weight loss (>5% of weight loss during the 6 months prior to surgery) was found to be as a reliable marker for malnutrition as SGA, MUST and NRS, whilst a low BMI was not [243, 246].

5.3.1. The obesity-paradox

A high BMI is associated with better outcome in cancer patients [247], which is often referred to as the obesity-paradox. However, recent studies investigated the hypothesis that adipose tissue may only have a protective effect in case of abundant muscle tissue, which is often the case in obesity. In order to do so, muscle mass, fat mass and BMI were measured in patients undergoing surgery for a malignancy. Indeed, a high BMI (>25) was associated with a longer overall survival. However, the shortest survival was observed in patients with a relatively high BMI but with a low muscle mass, i.e. in patients with sarcopenic obesity [248].

6. Conclusion

Surgery for cancer of the alimentary tract involves extensive and complex procedures. These surgical procedures have improved in the last decades; new techniques and treatment options have broadened the field of surgical oncology for abdominal cancers. Despite this improve-

http://dx.doi.org/10.5772/64775

ment, the postoperative outcome, in terms of postoperative morbidity, remains a significant issue for the patient and the physician.

One of the biggest challenges, in regard to postoperative outcome, is the aging population that undergoes surgery for cancer. Functional compromise, defined by several conditions such as fatigue, sarcopenia, cachexia, malnutrition, the presence of comorbidities and frailty, is especially common in the elderly patient, making them more susceptible to surgical stressors. Several screening tools have been developed to assess the presence of these conditions in order to identify avoidable perioperative risks.

There is an increasing need for protocoled care and new care pathways to reduce perioperative morbidity. The introduction of fast-track and enhanced recovery programs has led to a faster patient recovery and a reduction of complications after abdominal surgery. These care programs are aimed at reducing the surgical stressors. General principles of such programs are: minimized preoperative fasting, limited use of incisions, catheters and drains, early resumption of diet and early mobilization after surgery and optimal pain control. In addition, every type of surgery has its specific recommendations for protocoled care.

A multimodal approach is recommended when planning surgery for a compromised patient, including control of chronic diseases, referral to a geriatric specialist and optimizing nutritional status and exercise tolerance. Cardiopulmonary exercise testing can be used before surgery to determine the patient's cardiorespiratory fitness. Subsequently, exercise interventions before treatment can be used in cancer patients with a poor cardiorespiratory fitness to improve the treatment results. Regarding the nutritional status, this can be compromised due to cancer-related anorexia and cachexia. Preoperative assessment of the nutritional status should be considered, as malnourishment can have a negative effect on the postoperative outcome.

Author details

Audrey C.H.M. Jongen†[1*], Victor van Woerden†[1], Jeroen L.A. van Vugt[2], Patrick A. de Hoogt[3], Elisabeth M.L. de Wijkerslooth de Weerdesteijn[3], Juul J.W. Tegels[3], Nicole D. Bouvy[3] and Jan H.M.B. Stoot[3]

*Address all correspondence to: a.jongen@maastrichtuniversity.nl

1 Department of Surgery, Maastricht University Medical Centre, Maastricht, The Netherlands

2 Department of Surgery, Erasmus University Medical Centre, Rotterdam, The Netherlands

3 Department of Surgery, Zuyderland Medical Centre, Sittard-Geleen, The Netherlands

† These authors contributed equally to this work

References

[1] Ferlay J, Soerjomataram I, Dikshit R, Eser S, Mathers C, Rebelo M, et al. Cancer incidence and mortality worldwide: sources, methods and major patterns in GLOBOCAN 2012. International Journal of Cancer (Journal international du cancer). 2015 Mar 1;136(5):E359–86. PubMed PMID: 25220842. Epub 2014/09/16.

[2] Jakobson T, Karjagin J, Vipp L, Padar M, Parik AH, Starkopf L, et al. Postoperative complications and mortality after major gastrointestinal surgery. Medicina. 2014;50(2): 111–7. PubMed PMID: 25172605. Epub 2014/06/24.

[3] Jemal A, Bray F, Center MM, Ferlay J, Ward E, Forman D. Global cancer statistics. CA: A Cancer Journal for Clinicians. 2011 Mar–Apr;61(2):69–90. PubMed PMID: 21296855. Epub 2011/02/08.

[4] Vlug MS, Wind J, Hollmann MW, Ubbink DT, Cense HA, Engel AF, et al. Laparoscopy in combination with fast track multimodal management is the best perioperative strategy in patients undergoing colonic surgery: a randomized clinical trial (LAFA-study). Annals of Surgery. 2011 Dec;254(6):868–75. PubMed PMID: 21597360.

[5] Roulin D, Donadini A, Gander S, Griesser AC, Blanc C, Hubner M, et al. Cost-effectiveness of the implementation of an enhanced recovery protocol for colorectal surgery. The British Journal of Surgery. 2013 Jul;100(8):1108–14. PubMed PMID: 23754650.

[6] Basse L, Jakobsen DH, Bardram L, Billesbolle P, Lund C, Mogensen T, et al. Functional recovery after open versus laparoscopic colonic resection: a randomized, blinded study. Annals of Surgery. 2005 Mar;241(3):416–23. PubMed PMID: 15729063. Pubmed Central PMCID: 1356979.

[7] van Vugt JL, Reisinger KW, Derikx JP, Boerma D, Stoot JH. Improving the outcomes in oncological colorectal surgery. World Journal of Gastroenterology: WJG. 2014 Sep 21;20(35):12445–57. PubMed PMID: 25253944. Pubmed Central PMCID: PMC4168077. Epub 2014/09/26. eng.

[8] Berrino F, Verdecchia A, Lutz JM, Lombardo C, Micheli A, Capocaccia R, et al. Comparative cancer survival information in Europe. European Journal of Cancer. 2009 Apr; 45(6):901–8. PubMed PMID: 19217771. Epub 2009/02/17.

[9] Protopapa KL, Simpson JC, Smith NC, Moonesinghe SR. Development and validation of the Surgical Outcome Risk Tool (SORT). The British Journal of Surgery. 2014 Dec; 101(13):1774–83. PubMed PMID: 25388883. Pubmed Central PMCID: 4240514.

[10] Cohen ME, Bilimoria KY, Ko CY, Hall BL. Development of an American College of Surgeons National Surgery Quality Improvement Program: morbidity and mortality risk calculator for colorectal surgery. Journal of the American College of Surgeons. 2009 Jun;208(6):1009–16. PubMed PMID: 19476884.

[11] Hamaker ME, Jonker JM, de Rooij SE, Vos AG, Smorenburg CH, van Munster BC. Frailty screening methods for predicting outcome of a comprehensive geriatric

assessment in elderly patients with cancer: a systematic review. The Lancet Oncology. 2012 Oct;13(10):e437–44. PubMed PMID: 23026829.

[12] Fried LP, Tangen CM, Walston J, Newman AB, Hirsch C, Gottdiener J, et al. Frailty in older adults: evidence for a phenotype. The Journals of Gerontology Series A, Biological Sciences and Medical Sciences. 2001 Mar;56(3):M146–56. PubMed PMID: 11253156.

[13] Soubeyran P, Fonck M, Blanc-Bisson C, Blanc JF, Ceccaldi J, Mertens C, et al. Predictors of early death risk in older patients treated with first-line chemotherapy for cancer. Journal of Clinical Oncology: Official Journal of the American Society of Clinical Oncology. 2012 May 20;30(15):1829–34. PubMed PMID: 22508806.

[14] Schuurmans H, Steverink N, Lindenberg S, Frieswijk N, Slaets JP. Old or frail: what tells us more? The Journals of Gerontology Series A, Biological Sciences and Medical Sciences. 2004 Sep;59(9):M962–5. PubMed PMID: 15472162.

[15] Kruizenga HM, Seidell JC, de Vet HC, Wierdsma NJ, van Bokhorst-de van der Schueren MA. Development and validation of a hospital screening tool for malnutrition: the short nutritional assessment questionnaire (SNAQ). Clinical Nutrition. 2005 Feb;24(1):75–82. PubMed PMID: 15681104.

[16] Rahman A, Wu T, Bricknell R, Muqtadir Z, Armstrong D. Malnutrition matters in Canadian hospitalized patients: malnutrition risk in hospitalized patients in a tertiary care center using the malnutrition universal screening tool. Nutrition in Clinical Practice: Official Publication of the American Society for Parenteral and Enteral Nutrition. 2015 Oct;30(5):709–13. PubMed PMID: 26253124.

[17] Pohl H, Sirovich B, Welch HG. Esophageal adenocarcinoma incidence: are we reaching the peak? Cancer Epidemiology, Biomarkers & Prevention: A Publication of the American Association for Cancer Research, cosponsored by the American Society of Preventive Oncology. 2010 Jun;19(6):1468–70. PubMed PMID: 20501776. Epub 2010/05/27.

[18] Buas MF, Vaughan TL. Epidemiology and risk factors for gastroesophageal junction tumors: understanding the rising incidence of this disease. Seminars in Radiation Oncology. 2013 Jan;23(1):3–9. PubMed PMID: 23207041. Pubmed Central PMCID: 3535292. Epub 2012/12/05.

[19] Edgren G, Adami HO, Weiderpass E, Nyren O. A global assessment of the oesophageal adenocarcinoma epidemic. Gut. 2013 Oct;62(10):1406–14. PubMed PMID: 22917659. Epub 2012/08/25.

[20] Bollschweiler E, Wolfgarten E, Gutschow C, Holscher AH. Demographic variations in the rising incidence of esophageal adenocarcinoma in white males. Cancer. 2001 Aug 1;92(3):549–55. PubMed PMID: 11505399. Epub 2001/08/16.

[21] Zhang ZF, Kurtz RC, Sun M, Karpeh M, Jr., Yu GP, Gargon N, et al. Adenocarcinomas of the esophagus and gastric cardia: medical conditions, tobacco, alcohol, and socioeconomic factors. Cancer Epidemiology, Biomarkers & Prevention: A Publication

of the American Association for Cancer Research, cosponsored by the American Society of Preventive Oncology. 1996 Oct;5(10):761–8. PubMed PMID: 8896886. Epub 1996/10/01.

[22] Zambon P, Talamini R, La Vecchia C, Dal Maso L, Negri E, Tognazzo S, et al. Smoking, type of alcoholic beverage and squamous-cell oesophageal cancer in northern Italy. International Journal of Cancer (Journal International du cancer). 2000 Apr 1;86(1):144–9. PubMed PMID: 10728609. Epub 2000/03/23.

[23] Launoy G, Milan C, Faivre J, Pienkowski P, Gignoux M. Tobacco type and risk of squamous cell cancer of the oesophagus in males: a French multicentre case-control study. International Journal of Epidemiology. 2000 Feb;29(1):36–42. PubMed PMID: 10750601. Epub 2000/04/06.

[24] Engel LS, Chow WH, Vaughan TL, Gammon MD, Risch HA, Stanford JL, et al. Population attributable risks of esophageal and gastric cancers. Journal of the National Cancer Institute. 2003 Sep 17;95(18):1404–13. PubMed PMID: 13130116. Epub 2003/09/18.

[25] Stahl M, Stuschke M, Lehmann N, Meyer HJ, Walz MK, Seeber S, et al. Chemoradiation with and without surgery in patients with locally advanced squamous cell carcinoma of the esophagus. Journal of Clinical Oncology: Official Journal of the American Society of Clinical Oncology. 2005 Apr 1;23(10):2310–7. PubMed PMID: 15800321. Epub 2005/04/01.

[26] Bedenne L, Michel P, Bouche O, Milan C, Mariette C, Conroy T, et al. Chemoradiation followed by surgery compared with chemoradiation alone in squamous cancer of the esophagus: FFCD 9102. Journal of Clinical Oncology: Official Journal of the American Society of Clinical Oncology. 2007 Apr 1;25(10):1160–8. PubMed PMID: 17401004. Epub 2007/04/03.

[27] Jin HL, Zhu H, Ling TS, Zhang HJ, Shi RH. Neoadjuvant chemoradiotherapy for resectable esophageal carcinoma: a meta-analysis. World Journal of Gastroenterology. 2009 Dec 21;15(47):5983–91. PubMed PMID: 20014464. Pubmed Central PMCID: 2795187. Epub 2009/12/17.

[28] Lv J, Cao XF, Zhu B, Ji L, Tao L, Wang DD. Long-term efficacy of perioperative chemoradiotherapy on esophageal squamous cell carcinoma. World Journal of Gastroenterology. 2010 Apr 7;16(13):1649–54. PubMed PMID: 20355244. Pubmed Central PMCID: 2848374. Epub 2010/04/01.

[29] van Hagen P, Hulshof MC, van Lanschot JJ, Steyerberg EW, van Berge Henegouwen MI, Wijnhoven BP, et al. Preoperative chemoradiotherapy for esophageal or junctional cancer. The New England Journal of Medicine. 2012 May 31;366(22):2074–84. PubMed PMID: 22646630. Epub 2012/06/01.

[30] Fiorica F, Di Bona D, Schepis F, Licata A, Shahied L, Venturi A, et al. Preoperative chemoradiotherapy for oesophageal cancer: a systematic review and meta-analysis.

Gut. 2004 Jul;53(7):925–30. PubMed PMID: 15194636. Pubmed Central PMCID: 1774092. Epub 2004/06/15.

[31] Kumar S, Dimri K, Khurana R, Rastogi N, Das KJ, Lal P. A randomised trial of radiotherapy compared with cisplatin chemo-radiotherapy in patients with unresectable squamous cell cancer of the esophagus. Radiotherapy and Oncology: Journal of the European Society for Therapeutic Radiology and Oncology. 2007 May;83(2):139–47. PubMed PMID: 17445928. Epub 2007/04/21.

[32] Cooper JS, Guo MD, Herskovic A, Macdonald JS, Martenson JA, Jr., Al-Sarraf M, et al. Chemoradiotherapy of locally advanced esophageal cancer: long-term follow-up of a prospective randomized trial (RTOG 85-01). Radiation Therapy Oncology Group. JAMA. 1999 May 5;281(17):1623–7. PubMed PMID: 10235156. Epub 1999/05/11.

[33] Wong R, Malthaner R. Combined chemotherapy and radiotherapy (without surgery) compared with radiotherapy alone in localized carcinoma of the esophagus. The Cochrane Database of Systematic Reviews. 2001 (2):CD002092. PubMed PMID: 11406033. Epub 2001/06/19.

[34] Solcia E, Fiocca R, Luinetti O, Villani L, Padovan L, Calistri D, et al. Intestinal and diffuse gastric cancers arise in a different background of Helicobacter pylori gastritis through different gene involvement. The American Journal of Surgical Pathology. 1996;20 Suppl 1:S8–22. PubMed PMID: 8694148. Epub 1996/01/01.

[35] Correa P. A human model of gastric carcinogenesis. Cancer Research. 1988 Jul 1;48(13): 3554–60. PubMed PMID: 3288329. Epub 1988/07/01.

[36] Tramacere I, Negri E, Pelucchi C, Bagnardi V, Rota M, Scotti L, et al. A meta-analysis on alcohol drinking and gastric cancer risk. Annals of Oncology: Official Journal of the European Society for Medical Oncology/ESMO. 2012 Jan;23(1):28–36. PubMed PMID: 21536659. Epub 2011/05/04.

[37] Ladeiras-Lopes R, Pereira AK, Nogueira A, Pinheiro-Torres T, Pinto I, Santos-Pereira R, et al. Smoking and gastric cancer: systematic review and meta-analysis of cohort studies. Cancer Causes & Control: CCC. 2008 Sep;19(7):689–701. PubMed PMID: 18293090. Epub 2008/02/23.

[38] Dicken BJ, Bigam DL, Cass C, Mackey JR, Joy AA, Hamilton SM. Gastric adenocarcinoma: review and considerations for future directions. Annals of Surgery. 2005 Jan; 241(1):27–39. PubMed PMID: 15621988. Pubmed Central PMCID: 1356843. Epub 2004/12/29.

[39] Haverkamp L, Brenkman HJ, Seesing MF, Gisbertz SS, van Berge Henegouwen MI, Luyer MD, et al. Laparoscopic versus open gastrectomy for gastric cancer, a multicenter prospectively randomized controlled trial (LOGICA-trial). BMC Cancer. 2015;15:556. PubMed PMID: 26219670. Pubmed Central PMCID: 4518687. Epub 2015/07/30.

[40] Wanebo HJ, Kennedy BJ, Chmiel J, Steele G, Jr., Winchester D, Osteen R. Cancer of the stomach. A patient care study by the American College of Surgeons. Annals of Surgery.

1993 Nov;218(5):583–92. PubMed PMID: 8239772. Pubmed Central PMCID: 1243028. Epub 1993/11/01.

[41] Chau I, Norman AR, Cunningham D, Waters JS, Oates J, Ross PJ. Multivariate prognostic factor analysis in locally advanced and metastatic esophago-gastric cancer--pooled analysis from three multicenter, randomized, controlled trials using individual patient data. Journal of Clinical Oncology: Official Journal of the American Society of Clinical Oncology. 2004 Jun 15;22(12):2395–403. PubMed PMID: 15197201. Epub 2004/06/16.

[42] Hartgrink HH, van de Velde CJ, Putter H, Bonenkamp JJ, Klein Kranenbarg E, Songun I, et al. Extended lymph node dissection for gastric cancer: who may benefit? Final results of the randomized Dutch gastric cancer group trial. Journal of Clinical Oncology: Official Journal of the American Society of Clinical Oncology. 2004 Jun 1;22(11): 2069–77. PubMed PMID: 15082726. Epub 2004/04/15.

[43] McCulloch P, Nita ME, Kazi H, Gama-Rodrigues J. Extended versus limited lymph nodes dissection technique for adenocarcinoma of the stomach. The Cochrane Database of Systematic Reviews. 2004 (4):CD001964. PubMed PMID: 15495024. Epub 2004/10/21.

[44] Cunningham D, Allum WH, Stenning SP, Thompson JN, Van de Velde CJ, Nicolson M, et al. Perioperative chemotherapy versus surgery alone for resectable gastroesophageal cancer. The New England Journal of Medicine. 2006 Jul 6;355(1):11–20. PubMed PMID: 16822992. Epub 2006/07/11.

[45] Ronellenfitsch U, Schwarzbach M, Hofheinz R, Kienle P, Kieser M, Slanger TE, et al. Perioperative chemo(radio)therapy versus primary surgery for resectable adenocarcinoma of the stomach, gastroesophageal junction, and lower esophagus. The Cochrane Database of Systematic Reviews. 2013;5:CD008107. PubMed PMID: 23728671. Epub 2013/06/04.

[46] European Association for the Study of the L, European Organisation For R, Treatment of C. EASL-EORTC clinical practice guidelines: management of hepatocellular carcinoma. Journal of Hepatology. 2012 Apr;56(4):908–43. PubMed PMID: 22424438. Epub 2012/03/20.

[47] Yang JD, Harmsen WS, Slettedahl SW, Chaiteerakij R, Enders FT, Therneau TM, et al. Factors that affect risk for hepatocellular carcinoma and effects of surveillance. Clinical Gastroenterology and Hepatology: The Official Clinical Practice Journal of the American Gastroenterological Association. 2011 Jul;9(7):617–23 e1. PubMed PMID: 21459158. Epub 2011/04/05.

[48] Bruix J, Sherman M, American Association for the Study of Liver D. Management of hepatocellular carcinoma: an update. Hepatology. 2011 Mar;53(3):1020–2. PubMed PMID: 21374666. Pubmed Central PMCID: 3084991. Epub 2011/03/05.

[49] Singal A, Volk ML, Waljee A, Salgia R, Higgins P, Rogers MA, et al. Meta-analysis: surveillance with ultrasound for early-stage hepatocellular carcinoma in patients with

cirrhosis. Alimentary Pharmacology & Therapeutics. 2009 Jul;30(1):37–47. PubMed PMID: 19392863. Epub 2009/04/28.

[50] Cho YK, Kim JK, Kim MY, Rhim H, Han JK. Systematic review of randomized trials for hepatocellular carcinoma treated with percutaneous ablation therapies. Hepatology. 2009 Feb;49(2):453–9. PubMed PMID: 19065676. Epub 2008/12/10.

[51] Tiong L, Maddern GJ. Systematic review and meta-analysis of survival and disease recurrence after radiofrequency ablation for hepatocellular carcinoma. The British Journal of Surgery. 2011 Sep;98(9):1210–24. PubMed PMID: 21766289. Epub 2011/07/19.

[52] Germani G, Pleguezuelo M, Gurusamy K, Meyer T, Isgro G, Burroughs AK. Clinical outcomes of radiofrequency ablation, percutaneous alcohol and acetic acid injection for hepatocelullar carcinoma: a meta-analysis. Journal of Hepatology. 2010 Mar;52(3):380–8. PubMed PMID: 20149473. Epub 2010/02/13.

[53] Llovet JM, Bruix J. Systematic review of randomized trials for unresectable hepatocellular carcinoma: chemoembolization improves survival. Hepatology. 2003 Feb;37(2): 429–42. PubMed PMID: 12540794. Epub 2003/01/24.

[54] Camma C, Schepis F, Orlando A, Albanese M, Shahied L, Trevisani F, et al. Transarterial chemoembolization for unresectable hepatocellular carcinoma: meta-analysis of randomized controlled trials. Radiology. 2002 Jul;224(1):47–54. PubMed PMID: 12091661. Epub 2002/07/02.

[55] Zhang T, Ding X, Wei D, Cheng P, Su X, Liu H, et al. Sorafenib improves the survival of patients with advanced hepatocellular carcinoma: a meta-analysis of randomized trials. Anti-cancer Drugs. 2010 Mar;21(3):326–32. PubMed PMID: 20016366. Epub 2009/12/18.

[56] Lynch SM, Vrieling A, Lubin JH, Kraft P, Mendelsohn JB, Hartge P, et al. Cigarette smoking and pancreatic cancer: a pooled analysis from the pancreatic cancer cohort consortium. American Journal of Epidemiology. 2009 Aug 15;170(4):403–13. PubMed PMID: 19561064. Pubmed Central PMCID: 2733861. Epub 2009/06/30.

[57] Bosetti C, Lucenteforte E, Silverman DT, Petersen G, Bracci PM, Ji BT, et al. Cigarette smoking and pancreatic cancer: an analysis from the International Pancreatic Cancer Case-Control Consortium (Panc4). Annals of Oncology: Official Journal of the European Society for Medical Oncology/ESMO. 2012 Jul;23(7): 1880–8. PubMed PMID: 22104574. Pubmed Central PMCID: 3387822. Epub 2011/11/23.

[58] Bang UC, Benfield T, Hyldstrup L, Bendtsen F, Beck Jensen JE. Mortality, cancer, and comorbidities associated with chronic pancreatitis: a Danish nationwide matched-cohort study. Gastroenterology. 2014 Apr;146(4):989–94. PubMed PMID: 24389306. Epub 2014/01/07.

[59] Duell EJ, Lucenteforte E, Olson SH, Bracci PM, Li D, Risch HA, et al. Pancreatitis and pancreatic cancer risk: a pooled analysis in the International Pancreatic Cancer Case-

Control Consortium (PanC4). Annals of Oncology: Official Journal of the European Society for Medical Oncology/ESMO. 2012 Nov;23(11):2964–70. PubMed PMID: 22767586. Pubmed Central PMCID: 3477881. Epub 2012/07/07.

[60] Arslan AA, Helzlsouer KJ, Kooperberg C, Shu XO, Steplowski E, Bueno-de-Mesquita HB, et al. Anthropometric measures, body mass index, and pancreatic cancer: a pooled analysis from the Pancreatic Cancer Cohort Consortium (PanScan). Archives of Internal Medicine. 2010 May 10;170(9):791–802. PubMed PMID: 20458087. Pubmed Central PMCID: 2920035. Epub 2010/05/12.

[61] Aune D, Greenwood DC, Chan DS, Vieira R, Vieira AR, Navarro Rosenblatt DA, et al. Body mass index, abdominal fatness and pancreatic cancer risk: a systematic review and non-linear dose-response meta-analysis of prospective studies. Annals of Oncology: Official Journal of the European Society for Medical Oncology/ESMO. 2012 Apr; 23(4):843–52. PubMed PMID: 21890910. Epub 2011/09/06.

[62] Jacobs EJ, Chanock SJ, Fuchs CS, Lacroix A, McWilliams RR, Steplowski E, et al. Family history of cancer and risk of pancreatic cancer: a pooled analysis from the Pancreatic Cancer Cohort Consortium (PanScan). International Journal of Cancer (Journal International du Cancer). 2010 Sep 1;127(6):1421–8. PubMed PMID: 20049842. Pubmed Central PMCID: 2926939. Epub 2010/01/06.

[63] Brune KA, Lau B, Palmisano E, Canto M, Goggins MG, Hruban RH, et al. Importance of age of onset in pancreatic cancer kindreds. Journal of the National Cancer Institute. 2010 Jan 20;102(2):119–26. PubMed PMID: 20068195. Pubmed Central PMCID: 2808346. Epub 2010/01/14.

[64] Schenk M, Schwartz AG, O'Neal E, Kinnard M, Greenson JK, Fryzek JP, et al. Familial risk of pancreatic cancer. Journal of the National Cancer Institute. 2001 Apr 18;93(8): 640–4. PubMed PMID: 11309441. Epub 2001/04/20.

[65] Mancuso A, Calabro F, Sternberg CN. Current therapies and advances in the treatment of pancreatic cancer. Critical reviews in oncology/hematology. 2006 Jun;58(3):231–41. PubMed PMID: 16725343. Epub 2006/05/27.

[66] Cameron JL, Riall TS, Coleman J, Belcher KA. One thousand consecutive pancreaticoduodenectomies. Annals of Surgery. 2006 Jul;244(1):10–5. PubMed PMID: 16794383. Pubmed Central PMCID: 1570590. Epub 2006/06/24.

[67] Geer RJ, Brennan MF. Prognostic indicators for survival after resection of pancreatic adenocarcinoma. American Journal of Surgery. 1993 Jan;165(1):68–72; discussion -3. PubMed PMID: 8380315. Epub 1993/01/01.

[68] Kang MJ, Jang JY, Chang YR, Kwon W, Jung W, Kim SW. Revisiting the concept of lymph node metastases of pancreatic head cancer: number of metastatic lymph nodes and lymph node ratio according to N stage. Annals of Surgical Oncology. 2014 May;21(5): 1545–51. PubMed PMID: 24419758. Epub 2014/01/15.

[69] Garcea G, Dennison AR, Pattenden CJ, Neal CP, Sutton CD, Berry DP. Survival following curative resection for pancreatic ductal adenocarcinoma. A systematic review of the literature. JOP: Journal of the Pancreas. 2008;9(2):99–132. PubMed PMID: 18326920. Epub 2008/03/11.

[70] Ueno H, Kosuge T, Matsuyama Y, Yamamoto J, Nakao A, Egawa S, et al. A randomised phase III trial comparing gemcitabine with surgery-only in patients with resected pancreatic cancer: Japanese Study Group of Adjuvant Therapy for Pancreatic Cancer. British Journal of Cancer. 2009 Sep 15;101(6):908–15. PubMed PMID: 19690548. Pubmed Central PMCID: 2743365. Epub 2009/08/20.

[71] Oettle H, Post S, Neuhaus P, Gellert K, Langrehr J, Ridwelski K, et al. Adjuvant chemotherapy with gemcitabine vs observation in patients undergoing curative-intent resection of pancreatic cancer: a randomized controlled trial. JAMA. 2007 Jan 17;297(3): 267–77. PubMed PMID: 17227978. Epub 2007/01/18.

[72] Neoptolemos JP, Stocken DD, Friess H, Bassi C, Dunn JA, Hickey H, et al. A randomized trial of chemoradiotherapy and chemotherapy after resection of pancreatic cancer. The New England Journal of Medicine. 2004 Mar 18;350(12):1200–10. PubMed PMID: 15028824. Epub 2004/03/19.

[73] Evans DB, Varadhachary GR, Crane CH, Sun CC, Lee JE, Pisters PW, et al. Preoperative gemcitabine-based chemoradiation for patients with resectable adenocarcinoma of the pancreatic head. Journal of Clinical Oncology: Official Journal of the American Society of Clinical Oncology. 2008 Jul 20;26(21):3496–502. PubMed PMID: 18640930. Epub 2008/07/22.

[74] Gillen S, Schuster T, Meyer Zum Buschenfelde C, Friess H, Kleeff J. Preoperative/ neoadjuvant therapy in pancreatic cancer: a systematic review and meta-analysis of response and resection percentages. PLoS Medicine. 2010 Apr;7(4):e1000267. PubMed PMID: 20422030. Pubmed Central PMCID: 2857873. Epub 2010/04/28.

[75] Quiros RM, Brown KM, Hoffman JP. Neoadjuvant therapy in pancreatic cancer. Cancer Investigation. 2007 Jun;25(4):267–73. PubMed PMID: 17612937. Epub 2007/07/07.

[76] Tinkl D, Grabenbauer GG, Golcher H, Meyer T, Papadopoulos T, Hohenberger W, et al. Downstaging of pancreatic carcinoma after neoadjuvant chemoradiation. Strahlentherapie und Onkologie: Organ der Deutschen Rontgengesellschaft [et al]. 2009 Sep; 185(9):557–66. PubMed PMID: 19756421. Epub 2009/09/17.

[77] Nieveen van Dijkum EJ, Romijn MG, Terwee CB, de Wit LT, van der Meulen JH, Lameris HS, et al. Laparoscopic staging and subsequent palliation in patients with peripancreatic carcinoma. Annals of Surgery. 2003 Jan;237(1):66–73. PubMed PMID: 12496532. Pubmed Central PMCID: 1513968. Epub 2002/12/24.

[78] Sultana A, Tudur Smith C, Cunningham D, Starling N, Neoptolemos JP, Ghaneh P. Meta-analyses of chemotherapy for locally advanced and metastatic pancreatic cancer:

results of secondary end points analyses. British Journal of Cancer. 2008 Jul 8;99(1):6–13. PubMed PMID: 18577990. Pubmed Central PMCID: 2453014. Epub 2008/06/26.

[79] Van Heek NT, De Castro SM, van Eijck CH, van Geenen RC, Hesselink EJ, Breslau PJ, et al. The need for a prophylactic gastrojejunostomy for unresectable periampullary cancer: a prospective randomized multicenter trial with special focus on assessment of quality of life. Annals of Surgery. 2003 Dec;238(6):894–902; discussion -5. PubMed PMID: 14631226. Pubmed Central PMCID: 1356171. Epub 2003/11/25.

[80] Yip D, Karapetis C, Strickland A, Steer CB, Goldstein D. Chemotherapy and radiotherapy for inoperable advanced pancreatic cancer. The Cochrane Database of Systematic Reviews. 2006 (3):CD002093. PubMed PMID: 16855985. Epub 2006/07/21.

[81] Cunningham D, Chau I, Stocken DD, Valle JW, Smith D, Steward W, et al. Phase III randomized comparison of gemcitabine versus gemcitabine plus capecitabine in patients with advanced pancreatic cancer. Journal of Clinical Oncology: Official Journal of the American Society of Clinical Oncology. 2009 Nov 20;27(33):5513–8. PubMed PMID: 19858379. Epub 2009/10/28.

[82] Duffy A, Capanu M, Abou-Alfa GK, Huitzil D, Jarnagin W, Fong Y, et al. Gallbladder cancer (GBC): 10-year experience at Memorial Sloan-Kettering Cancer Centre (MSKCC). Journal of Surgical Oncology. 2008 Dec 1;98(7):485–9. PubMed PMID: 18802958. Epub 2008/09/20.

[83] Konstantinidis IT, Deshpande V, Genevay M, Berger D, Fernandez-del Castillo C, Tanabe KK, et al. Trends in presentation and survival for gallbladder cancer during a period of more than 4 decades: a single-institution experience. Archives of Surgery. 2009 May;144(5):441–7; discussion 7. PubMed PMID: 19451486. Epub 2009/05/20.

[84] van Gulik TM, Gouma DJ. Changing perspectives in the assessment of resectability of hilar cholangiocarcinoma. Annals of Surgical Oncology. 2007 Jul;14(7):1969–71. PubMed PMID: 17453297. Pubmed Central PMCID: 1914233. Epub 2007/04/25.

[85] van Gulik TM, Kloek JJ, Ruys AT, Busch OR, van Tienhoven GJ, Lameris JS, et al. Multidisciplinary management of hilar cholangiocarcinoma (Klatskin tumor): extended resection is associated with improved survival. European Journal of Surgical Oncology: The Journal of the European Society of Surgical Oncology and the British Association of Surgical Oncology. 2011 Jan;37(1):65–71. PubMed PMID: 21115233. Epub 2010/12/01.

[86] Hueman MT, Vollmer CM, Jr., Pawlik TM. Evolving treatment strategies for gallbladder cancer. Annals of Surgical Oncology. 2009 Aug;16(8):2101–15. PubMed PMID: 19495882. Epub 2009/06/06.

[87] Lai CH, Lau WY. Gallbladder cancer-—a comprehensive review. The Surgeon: Journal of the Royal Colleges of Surgeons of Edinburgh and Ireland. 2008 Apr;6(2):101–10. PubMed PMID: 18488776. Epub 2008/05/21.

[88] Gourgiotis S, Kocher HM, Solaini L, Yarollahi A, Tsiambas E, Salemis NS. Gallbladder cancer. American Journal of Surgery. 2008 Aug;196(2):252–64. PubMed PMID: 18466866. Epub 2008/05/10.

[89] Baton O, Azoulay D, Adam DV, Castaing D. Major hepatectomy for hilar cholangiocarcinoma type 3 and 4: prognostic factors and longterm outcomes. Journal of the American College of Surgeons. 2007 Feb;204(2):250–60. PubMed PMID: 17254929. Epub 2007/01/27.

[90] Kloek JJ, Ten Kate FJ, Busch OR, Gouma DJ, van Gulik TM. Surgery for extrahepatic cholangiocarcinoma: predictors of survival. HPB: The Official Journal of the International Hepato Pancreato Biliary Association. 2008;10(3):190–5. PubMed PMID: 18773053. Pubmed Central PMCID: 2504374. Epub 2008/09/06.

[91] Nimura Y. Preoperative biliary drainage before resection for cholangiocarcinoma (Pro). HPB: the official journal of the International Hepato Pancreato Biliary Association. 2008;10(2):130–3. PubMed PMID: 18773090. Pubmed Central PMCID: 2504393. Epub 2008/09/06.

[92] van der Gaag NA, Kloek JJ, de Castro SM, Busch OR, van Gulik TM, Gouma DJ. Preoperative biliary drainage in patients with obstructive jaundice: history and current status. Journal of Gastrointestinal Surgery: Official Journal of the Society for Surgery of the Alimentary Tract. 2009 Apr;13(4):814–20. PubMed PMID: 18726134. Epub 2008/08/30.

[93] Ebata T, Yokoyama Y, Igami T, Sugawara G, Takahashi Y, Nagino M. Portal vein embolization before extended hepatectomy for biliary cancer: current technique and review of 494 consecutive embolizations. Digestive Surgery. 2012;29(1):23–9. PubMed PMID: 22441616. Epub 2012/03/24.

[94] Nagino M, Kamiya J, Nishio H, Ebata T, Arai T, Nimura Y. Two hundred forty consecutive portal vein embolizations before extended hepatectomy for biliary cancer: surgical outcome and long-term follow-up. Annals of Surgery. 2006 Mar;243(3):364–72. PubMed PMID: 16495702. Pubmed Central PMCID: 1448943. Epub 2006/02/24.

[95] Horgan AM, Amir E, Walter T, Knox JJ. Adjuvant therapy in the treatment of biliary tract cancer: a systematic review and meta-analysis. Journal of Clinical Oncology: Official Journal of the American Society of Clinical Oncology. 2012 Jun 1;30(16):1934–40. PubMed PMID: 22529261. Epub 2012/04/25.

[96] Anderson C, Kim R. Adjuvant therapy for resected extrahepatic cholangiocarcinoma: a review of the literature and future directions. Cancer Treatment Reviews. 2009 Jun; 35(4):322–7. PubMed PMID: 19147294. Epub 2009/01/17.

[97] Skipworth JR, Olde Damink SW, Imber C, Bridgewater J, Pereira SP, Malago M. Review article: surgical, neo-adjuvant and adjuvant management strategies in biliary tract cancer. Alimentary Pharmacology & Therapeutics. 2011 Nov;34(9):1063–78. PubMed PMID: 21933219. Pubmed Central PMCID: 3235953. Epub 2011/09/22.

[98] Zauber AG, Winawer SJ, O'Brien MJ, Lansdorp-Vogelaar I, van Ballegooijen M, Hankey BF, et al. Colonoscopic polypectomy and long-term prevention of colorectal-cancer deaths. The New England Journal of Medicine. 2012 Feb 23;366(8):687–96. PubMed PMID: 22356322. Pubmed Central PMCID: 3322371. Epub 2012/02/24.

[99] Kohler BA, Sherman RL, Howlader N, Jemal A, Ryerson AB, Henry KA, et al. Annual report to the nation on the status of cancer, 1975–2011, featuring incidence of breast cancer subtypes by race/ethnicity, poverty, and state. Journal of the National Cancer Institute. 2015 Jun;107(6):djv048. PubMed PMID: 25825511. Pubmed Central PMCID: 4603551. Epub 2015/04/01.

[100] Atkin W, Dadswell E, Wooldrage K, Kralj-Hans I, von Wagner C, Edwards R, et al. Computed tomographic colonography versus colonoscopy for investigation of patients with symptoms suggestive of colorectal cancer (SIGGAR): a multicentre randomised trial. Lancet. 2013 Apr 6;381(9873):1194–202. PubMed PMID: 23414650. Epub 2013/02/19.

[101] Chan AT, Giovannucci EL. Primary prevention of colorectal cancer. Gastroenterology. 2010 Jun;138(6):2029–43 e10. PubMed PMID: 20420944. Pubmed Central PMCID: 2947820. Epub 2010/04/28.

[102] Rutter MD. Surveillance programmes for neoplasia in colitis. Journal of Gastroenterology. 2011 Jan;46 Suppl 1:1–5. PubMed PMID: 20798970. Epub 2010/08/28.

[103] Henderson TO, Oeffinger KC, Whitton J, Leisenring W, Neglia J, Meadows A, et al. Secondary gastrointestinal cancer in childhood cancer survivors: a cohort study. Annals of Internal Medicine. 2012 Jun 5;156(11):757–66, W-260. PubMed PMID: 22665813. Pubmed Central PMCID: 3554254. Epub 2012/06/06.

[104] Karahalios A, English DR, Simpson JA. Weight change and risk of colorectal cancer: a systematic review and meta-analysis. American Journal of Epidemiology. 2015 Jun 1;181(11):832–45. PubMed PMID: 25888582. Epub 2015/04/19.

[105] Chan DS, Lau R, Aune D, Vieira R, Greenwood DC, Kampman E, et al. Red and processed meat and colorectal cancer incidence: meta-analysis of prospective studies. PLoS One. 2011;6(6):e20456. PubMed PMID: 21674008. Pubmed Central PMCID: 3108955. Epub 2011/06/16.

[106] Botteri E, Iodice S, Bagnardi V, Raimondi S, Lowenfels AB, Maisonneuve P. Smoking and colorectal cancer: a meta-analysis. JAMA. 2008 Dec 17;300(23):2765–78. PubMed PMID: 19088354. Epub 2008/12/18.

[107] Weiss JM, Pfau PR, O'Connor ES, King J, LoConte N, Kennedy G, et al. Mortality by stage for right- versus left-sided colon cancer: analysis of surveillance, epidemiology, and end results—medicare data. Journal of Clinical Oncology: Official Journal of the American Society of Clinical Oncology. 2011 Nov 20;29(33):4401–9. PubMed PMID: 21969498. Pubmed Central PMCID: 3221523. Epub 2011/10/05.

[108] Cukier M, Smith AJ, Milot L, Chu W, Chung H, Fenech D, et al. Neoadjuvant chemoradiotherapy and multivisceral resection for primary locally advanced adherent colon cancer: a single institution experience. European Journal of Surgical Oncology: The Journal of the European Society of Surgical Oncology and the British Association of Surgical Oncology. 2012 Aug;38(8):677–82. PubMed PMID: 22632848. Epub 2012/05/29.

[109] Govindarajan A, Fraser N, Cranford V, Wirtzfeld D, Gallinger S, Law CH, et al. Predictors of multivisceral resection in patients with locally advanced colorectal cancer. Annals of Surgical Oncology. 2008 Jul;15(7):1923–30. PubMed PMID: 18473145. Pubmed Central PMCID: 2770244. Epub 2008/05/14.

[110] Audisio RA, Ramesh H, Longo WE, Zbar AP, Pope D. Preoperative assessment of surgical risk in oncogeriatric patients. Oncologist. 2005 Apr;10(4):262–8. PubMed PMID: 15821246.

[111] Polanczyk CA, Marcantonio E, Goldman L, Rohde LE, Orav J, Mangione CM, et al. Impact of age on perioperative complications and length of stay in patients undergoing noncardiac surgery. Annals of Internal Medicine. 2001 Apr 17;134(8):637–43. PubMed PMID: 11304103.

[112] Hamel MB, Henderson WG, Khuri SF, Daley J. Surgical outcomes for patients aged 80 and older: morbidity and mortality from major noncardiac surgery. Journal of the American Geriatrics Society. 2005 Mar;53(3):424–9. PubMed PMID: 15743284.

[113] Colorectal Cancer Collaborative Group. Surgery for colorectal cancer in elderly patients: a systematic review. Lancet. 2000 Sep 16;356(9234):968–74. PubMed PMID: 11041397.

[114] Blommers E, Klimek M, Hartholt KA, van der Cammen TJ, Klein J, Noordzij PG. Perioperative care of the older patient. Zeitschrift für Gerontologie und Geriatrie. 2011 Jun;44(3):187–91. PubMed PMID: 21607796.

[115] Charlson ME, Pompei P, Ales KL, MacKenzie CR. A new method of classifying prognostic comorbidity in longitudinal studies: development and validation. Journal of Chronic Diseases. 1987;40(5):373–83. PubMed PMID: 3558716. Pubmed Central PMCID: 3558716.

[116] Daabiss M. American Society of Anaesthesiologists physical status classification. Indian Journal of Anaesthesia. 2011 Mar;55(2):111–5. PubMed PMID: 21712864.

[117] Oken MM, Creech RH, Tormey DC, Horton J, Davis TE, McFadden ET, et al. Toxicity and response criteria of the Eastern Cooperative Oncology Group. American Journal of Clinical Oncology. 1982 Dec;5(6):649–55. PubMed PMID: 7165009.

[118] Makary MA, Segev DL, Pronovost PJ, Syin D, Bandeen-Roche K, Patel P, et al. Frailty as a predictor of surgical outcomes in older patients. Journal of the American College of Surgeons. 2010 Jun;210(6):901–8. PubMed PMID: 20510798.

[119] Mak PH, Campbell RC, Irwin MG, American Society of A. The ASA Physical Status Classification: inter-observer consistency. American Society of Anesthesiologists. Anaesthesia and Intensive Care. 2002 Oct;30(5):633–40. PubMed PMID: 12413266.

[120] Robinson TN, Eiseman B, Wallace JI, Church SD, McFann KK, Pfister SM, et al. Redefining geriatric preoperative assessment using frailty, disability and co-morbidity. Annals of Surgery. 2009 Sep;250(3):449–55. PubMed PMID: 19730176. Pubmed Central PMCID: 19730176.

[121] Dasgupta M, Rolfson DB, Stolee P, Borrie MJ, Speechley M. Frailty is associated with postoperative complications in older adults with medical problems. Archives of Gerontology and Geriatrics. 2009 Jan–Feb;48(1):78–83. PubMed PMID: 18068828. Pubmed Central PMCID: 18068828.

[122] Saxton A, Velanovich V. Preoperative frailty and quality of life as predictors of post-operative complications. Annals of Surgery. 2011 Jun;253(6):1223–9. PubMed PMID: 21412145.

[123] Roubenoff R. Sarcopenia: a major modifiable cause of frailty in the elderly. The Journal of Nutrition, Health and Aging. 2000;4(3):140–2. PubMed PMID: 10936900.

[124] Cooper C, Dere W, Evans W, Kanis JA, Rizzoli R, Sayer AA, et al. Frailty and sarcopenia: definitions and outcome parameters. Osteoporosis International. 2012 Jul;23(7):1839–48. PubMed PMID: 22290243.

[125] Marzetti E, Leeuwenburgh C. Skeletal muscle apoptosis, sarcopenia and frailty at old age. Experimental Gerontology. 2006 Dec;41(12):1234–8. PubMed PMID: 17052879.

[126] Cherin P, Voronska E, Fraoucene N, de Jaeger C. Prevalence of sarcopenia among healthy ambulatory subjects: the sarcopenia begins from 45 years. Aging clinical and experimental research. 2014 Apr;26(2):137–46. PubMed PMID: 24129803.

[127] Cruz-Jentoft AJ, Baeyens JP, Bauer JM, Boirie Y, Cederholm T, Landi F, et al. Sarcopenia: European consensus on definition and diagnosis: report of the European Working Group on Sarcopenia in Older People. Age and Ageing. 2010 Jul;39(4):412–23. PubMed PMID: 20392703. Pubmed Central PMCID: PMC2886201.

[128] Baumgartner RN, Koehler KM, Gallagher D, Romero L, Heymsfield SB, Ross RR, et al. Epidemiology of sarcopenia among the elderly in New Mexico. American Journal of Epidemiology. 1998 Apr 15;147(8):755–63. PubMed PMID: 9554417.

[129] Janssen I, Heymsfield SB, Ross R. Low relative skeletal muscle mass (sarcopenia) in older persons is associated with functional impairment and physical disability. Journal of the American Geriatrics Society. 2002 May;50(5):889–96. PubMed PMID: 12028177.

[130] Peng PD, van Vledder MG, Tsai S, de Jong MC, Makary M, Ng J, et al. Sarcopenia negatively impacts short-term outcomes in patients undergoing hepatic resection for colorectal liver metastasis. HPB : the official journal of the International Hepato

Pancreato Biliary Association. 2011 Jul;13(7):439–46. PubMed PMID: 21689226. Pubmed Central PMCID: 3133709.

[131] Peng P, Hyder O, Firoozmand A, Kneuertz P, Schulick RD, Huang D, et al. Impact of sarcopenia on outcomes following resection of pancreatic adenocarcinoma. Journal of Gastrointestinal Surgery. 2012 Aug;16(8):1478–86. PubMed PMID: 22692586. Pubmed Central PMCID: 3578313. Epub 2012/06/14. eng.

[132] van Vledder MG, Levolger S, Ayez N, Verhoef C, Tran TC, Ijzermans JN. Body composition and outcome in patients undergoing resection of colorectal liver metastases. British Journal of Surgery. 2012 Apr;99(4):550–7. PubMed PMID: 22246799. Epub 2012/01/17. eng.

[133] Tegels JJ, van Vugt JL, Reisinger KW, Hulsewe KW, Hoofwijk AG, Derikx JP, et al. Sarcopenia is highly prevalent in patients undergoing surgery for gastric cancer but not associated with worse outcomes. Journal of Surgical Oncology. 2015 Sep;112(4):403–7. PubMed PMID: 26331988.

[134] Wang SL, Zhuang CL, Huang DD, Pang WY, Lou N, Chen FF, et al. Sarcopenia adversely impacts postoperative clinical outcomes following gastrectomy in patients with gastric cancer: a prospective study. Annals of Surgical Oncology. 2015 Dec 14. PubMed PMID: 26668085.

[135] Fearon KC. Cancer cachexia: developing multimodal therapy for a multidimensional problem. European Journal of Cancer. 2008 May;44(8):1124–32. PubMed PMID: 18375115.

[136] Tisdale MJ. Mechanisms of cancer cachexia. Physiological Reviews. 2009 Apr;89(2):381–410. PubMed PMID: 19342610.

[137] Evans WJ, Morley JE, Argiles J, Bales C, Baracos V, Guttridge D, et al. Cachexia: a new definition. Clinical Nutrition. 2008 Dec;27(6):793–9. PubMed PMID: 18718696.

[138] Fearon K, Strasser F, Anker SD, Bosaeus I, Bruera E, Fainsinger RL, et al. Definition and classification of cancer cachexia: an international consensus. The Lancet Oncology. 2011 May;12(5):489–95. PubMed PMID: 21296615.

[139] Rolland Y, Abellan van Kan G, Gillette-Guyonnet S, Vellas B. Cachexia versus sarcopenia. Current Opinion in Clinical Nutrition and Metabolic Care. 2011 Jan;14(1):15–21. PubMed PMID: 21076295.

[140] Valle J, Wasan H, Palmer DH, Cunningham D, Anthoney A, Maraveyas A, et al. Cisplatin plus gemcitabine versus gemcitabine for biliary tract cancer. New England Journal of Medicine. 2010 Apr 8;362(14):1273–81. PubMed PMID: 20375404.

[141] Reisinger KW, Bosmans JW, Uittenbogaart M, Alsoumali A, Poeze M, Sosef MN, et al. Loss of skeletal muscle mass during neoadjuvant chemoradiotherapy predicts postoperative mortality in esophageal cancer surgery. Annals of Surgical Oncology. 2015 Apr 17. PubMed PMID: 25893413.

[142] Awad S, Tan BH, Cui H, Bhalla A, Fearon KC, Parsons SL, et al. Marked changes in body composition following neoadjuvant chemotherapy for oesophagogastric cancer. Clinical Nutrition. 2012 Feb;31(1):74–7. PubMed PMID: 21875767.

[143] Yip C, Goh V, Davies A, Gossage J, Mitchell-Hay R, Hynes O, et al. Assessment of sarcopenia and changes in body composition after neoadjuvant chemotherapy and associations with clinical outcomes in oesophageal cancer. European Radiology. 2014 May;24(5):998–1005. PubMed PMID: 24535076.

[144] Del Fabbro E, Parsons H, Warneke CL, Pulivarthi K, Litton JK, Dev R, et al. The relationship between body composition and response to neoadjuvant chemotherapy in women with operable breast cancer. Oncologist. 2012;17(10):1240–5. PubMed PMID: 22903527.

[145] Cooper AB, Slack R, Fogelman D, Holmes HM, Petzel M, Parker N, et al. Characterization of anthropometric changes that occur during neoadjuvant therapy for potentially resectable pancreatic cancer. Annals of Surgical Oncology. 2015 Jul;22(7):2416–23. PubMed PMID: 25519927.

[146] Dalal S, Hui D, Bidaut L, Lem K, Del Fabbro E, Crane C, et al. Relationships among body mass index, longitudinal body composition alterations, and survival in patients with locally advanced pancreatic cancer receiving chemoradiation: a pilot study. Journal of Pain and Symptom Management. 2012 Aug;44(2):181–91. PubMed PMID: 22695045.

[147] Ali R, Baracos VE, Sawyer MB, Bianchi L, Roberts S, Assenat E, et al. Lean body mass as an independent determinant of dose-limiting toxicity and neuropathy in patients with colon cancer treated with FOLFOX regimens. Cancer Medicine. 2016 Jan 27. PubMed PMID: 26814378.

[148] Antoun S, Borget I, Lanoy E. Impact of sarcopenia on the prognosis and treatment toxicities in patients diagnosed with cancer. Current Opinion in Supportive and Palliative Care. 2013 Dec;7(4):383–9. PubMed PMID: 24189893.

[149] Cousin S, Hollebecque A, Koscielny S, Mir O, Varga A, Baracos VE, et al. Low skeletal muscle is associated with toxicity in patients included in phase I trials. Investigational New Drugs. 2014 Apr;32(2):382–7. PubMed PMID: 24343673.

[150] Cushen SJ, Power DG, Teo MY, Maceneaney P, Maher MM, McDermott R, et al. Body composition by computed tomography as a predictor of toxicity in patients with renal cell carcinoma treated with sunitinib. American Journal of Clinical Oncology. 2014 Apr 21. PubMed PMID: 24685884.

[151] Prado CM, Baracos VE, McCargar LJ, Mourtzakis M, Mulder KE, Reiman T, et al. Body composition as an independent determinant of 5-fluorouracil-based chemotherapy toxicity. Clinical Cancer Research. 2007 Jun 1;13(11):3264–8. PubMed PMID: 17545532.

[152] Prado CM, Lima IS, Baracos VE, Bies RR, McCargar LJ, Reiman T, et al. An exploratory study of body composition as a determinant of epirubicin pharmacokinetics and toxicity. Cancer Chemotherapy and Pharmacology. 2011 Jan;67(1):93–101. PubMed PMID: 20204364.

[153] Tan BH, Brammer K, Randhawa N, Welch NT, Parsons SL, James EJ, et al. Sarcopenia is associated with toxicity in patients undergoing neo-adjuvant chemotherapy for oesophago-gastric cancer. European Journal of Surgical Oncology. 2015 Mar;41(3):333–8. PubMed PMID: 25498359.

[154] Fitz-Henry J. The ASA classification and peri-operative risk. Annals of the Royal College of Surgeons of England. 2011 Apr;93(3):185–7. PubMed PMID: 21477427. Pubmed Central PMCID: 3348554.

[155] Fujiwara Y, Tsujie M, Hara J, Kato H, Kitani K, Isono S, et al. Comparison of gastric cancer surgery between patients aged >80 years and <79 years: complications and multivariate analysis of prognostic factors. Hepato-gastroenterology. 2014 Sep;61(134): 1785–93. PubMed PMID: 25513165. Pubmed Central PMCID: 25436380.

[156] Takeshita H, Ichikawa D, Komatsu S, Kubota T, Okamoto K, Shiozaki A, et al. Surgical outcomes of gastrectomy for elderly patients with gastric cancer. World Journal of Surgery. 2013 Dec;37(12):2891–8. PubMed PMID: 24081528.

[157] Grendar J, Shaheen AA, Myers RP, Parker R, Vollmer CM, Jr., Ball CG, et al. Predicting in-hospital mortality in patients undergoing complex gastrointestinal surgery: determining the optimal risk adjustment method. Archives of Surgery. 2012 Feb;147(2):126–35. PubMed PMID: 22006854. Epub 2011/10/19. eng.

[158] Hsu JT, Liu MS, Wang F, Chang CJ, Hwang TL, Jan YY, et al. Standard radical gastrectomy in octogenarians and nonagenarians with gastric cancer: are short-term surgical results and long-term survival substantial? Journal of Gastrointestinal Surgery. 2012 Apr;16(4):728–37. PubMed PMID: 22350724. Pubmed Central PMCID: 22350724.

[159] Hoogendijk EO, van der Horst HE, Deeg DJ, Frijters DH, Prins BA, Jansen AP, et al. The identification of frail older adults in primary care: comparing the accuracy of five simple instruments. Age and Ageing. 2013 Mar;42(2):262–5. PubMed PMID: 23108163. Epub 2012/10/31. eng.

[160] Tegels JJ, de Maat MF, Hulsewe KW, Hoofwijk AG, Stoot JH. Value of geriatric frailty and nutritional status assessment in predicting postoperative mortality in gastric cancer surgery. Journal of Gastrointestinal Surgery. 2014 Mar;18(3):439–45; discussion 45–6. PubMed PMID: 24420730.

[161] Ommundsen N, Wyller TB, Nesbakken A, Jordhoy MS, Bakka A, Skovlund E, et al. Frailty is an independent predictor of survival in older patients with colorectal cancer. Oncologist. 2014 Dec;19(12):1268–75. PubMed PMID: 25355846. Pubmed Central PMCID: PMC4257747.

[162] Mariette C, De Botton ML, Piessen G. Surgery in esophageal and gastric cancer patients: what is the role for nutrition support in your daily practice? Annals of Surgical Oncology. 2012 Jul;19(7):2128–34. PubMed PMID: 22322948.

[163] Morley JE. Sarcopenia in the elderly. Family Practice. 2012 Apr;29 Suppl 1:i44–i8. PubMed PMID: 22399555.

[164] Martin L, Birdsell L, Macdonald N, Reiman T, Clandinin MT, McCargar LJ, et al. Cancer cachexia in the age of obesity: skeletal muscle depletion is a powerful prognostic factor, independent of body mass index. Journal of Clinical Oncology: Official Journal of the American Society of Clinical Oncology. 2013 Apr 20;31(12):1539–47. PubMed PMID: 23530101.

[165] Ryu SW, Kim IH. Comparison of different nutritional assessments in detecting malnutrition among gastric cancer patients. World Journal of Gastroenterology: WJG. 2010 Jul 14;16(26):3310–7. PubMed PMID: 20614488. Pubmed Central PMCID: PMC2900724.

[166] Bo Y, Yao M, Zhang L, Bekalo W, Lu W, Lu Q. Preoperative Nutritional Risk Index to predict postoperative survival time in primary liver cancer patients. Asia Pacific Journal of Clinical Nutrition. 2015;24(4):591–7. PubMed PMID: 26693742.

[167] Probst P, Haller S, Dorr-Harim C, Bruckner T, Ulrich A, Hackert T, et al. Nutritional risk in major abdominal surgery: protocol of a prospective observational trial to evaluate the prognostic value of different nutritional scores in pancreatic surgery. JMIR Research Protocols. 2015;4(4):e132. PubMed PMID: 26573991. Pubmed Central PMCID: PMC4704883.

[168] Kondrup J, Allison SP, Elia M, Vellas B, Plauth M, Educational, et al. ESPEN guidelines for nutrition screening 2002. Clinical Nutrition. 2003 Aug;22(4):415–21. PubMed PMID: 12880610.

[169] Webster S, Fletcher SJ. Fit for surgery? Preoperative assessment. Surgery – Oxford International Edition. 29(3):112–4.

[170] Fearon KC, Ljungqvist O, Von Meyenfeldt M, Revhaug A, Dejong CH, Lassen K, et al. Enhanced recovery after surgery: a consensus review of clinical care for patients undergoing colonic resection. Clinical Nutrition. 2005 Jun;24(3):466–77. PubMed PMID: 15896435.

[171] Kehlet H, Wilmore DW. Fast-track surgery. The British Journal of Surgery. 2005 Jan; 92(1):3–4. PubMed PMID: 15635603.

[172] Wilmore DW. From Cuthbertson to fast-track surgery: 70 years of progress in reducing stress in surgical patients. Annals of Surgery. 2002 Nov;236(5):643–8. PubMed PMID: 12409671. Pubmed Central PMCID: 1422623.

[173] Gustafsson UO, Scott MJ, Schwenk W, Demartines N, Roulin D, Francis N, et al. Guidelines for perioperative care in elective colonic surgery: Enhanced Recovery After

Surgery (ERAS((R))) Society recommendations. World Journal of Surgery. 2013 Feb; 37(2):259–84. PubMed PMID: 23052794.

[174] Feldheiser A, Aziz O, Baldini G, Cox BP, Fearon KC, Feldman LS, et al. Enhanced Recovery After Surgery (ERAS) for gastrointestinal surgery, part 2: consensus statement for anaesthesia practice. Acta Anaesthesiologica Scandinavica. 2016 Mar;60(3): 289–334. PubMed PMID: 26514824.

[175] Kehlet H, Wilmore DW. Multimodal strategies to improve surgical outcome. American Journal of Surgery. 2002 Jun;183(6):630–41. PubMed PMID: 12095591.

[176] Lassen K, Coolsen MM, Slim K, Carli F, de Aguilar-Nascimento JE, Schafer M, et al. Guidelines for perioperative care for pancreaticoduodenectomy: Enhanced Recovery After Surgery (ERAS(R)) Society recommendations. Clinical Nutrition. 2012 Dec;31(6): 817–30. PubMed PMID: 23079762.

[177] Nygren J, Thacker J, Carli F, Fearon KC, Norderval S, Lobo DN, et al. Guidelines for perioperative care in elective rectal/pelvic surgery: Enhanced Recovery After Surgery (ERAS((R))) Society recommendations. World Journal of Surgery. 2013 Feb;37(2):285–305. PubMed PMID: 23052796.

[178] Mortensen K, Nilsson M, Slim K, Schafer M, Mariette C, Braga M, et al. Consensus guidelines for enhanced recovery after gastrectomy: Enhanced Recovery After Surgery (ERAS(R)) Society recommendations. British Journal of Surgery. 2014 Sep;101(10):1209–29. PubMed PMID: 25047143.

[179] Wu SJ, Xiong XZ, Lu J, Cheng Y, Lin YX, Zhou RX, et al. Fast-track programs for liver surgery: a meta-analysis. Journal of Gastrointestinal Surgery. 2015 Jul 10. PubMed PMID: 26160321. Epub 2015/07/15. Eng.

[180] Hall TC, Dennison AR, Bilku DK, Metcalfe MS, Garcea G. Enhanced recovery programmes in hepatobiliary and pancreatic surgery: a systematic review. Annals of the Royal College of Surgeons of England. 2012 Jul;94(5):318–26. PubMed PMID: 22943226. Pubmed Central PMCID: PMC3954372. Epub 2012/09/05. eng.

[181] Spanjersberg WR, Reurings J, Keus F, van Laarhoven CJ. Fast track surgery versus conventional recovery strategies for colorectal surgery. The Cochrane Database of Systematic Reviews. 2011 (2):CD007635. PubMed PMID: 21328298.

[182] Grotenhuis BA, Wijnhoven BP, Grune F, van Bommel J, Tilanus HW, van Lanschot JJ. Preoperative risk assessment and prevention of complications in patients with esophageal cancer. Journal of Surgical Oncology. 2010 Mar 1;101(3):270–8. PubMed PMID: 20082349.

[183] van Stijn MF, Korkic-Halilovic I, Bakker MS, van der Ploeg T, van Leeuwen PA, Houdijk AP. Preoperative nutrition status and postoperative outcome in elderly general surgery patients: a systematic review. JPEN Journal of Parenteral and Enteral Nutrition. 2013 Jan;37(1):37–43. PubMed PMID: 22549764.

[184] Sultan J, Griffin SM, Di Franco F, Kirby JA, Shenton BK, Seal CJ, et al. Randomized clinical trial of omega-3 fatty acid-supplemented enteral nutrition versus standard enteral nutrition in patients undergoing oesophagogastric cancer surgery. British Journal of Surgery. 2012 Mar;99(3):346–55. PubMed PMID: 22237467. Pubmed Central PMCID: PMC3625735.

[185] Findlay JM, Gillies RS, Millo J, Sgromo B, Marshall RE, Maynard ND. Enhanced recovery for esophagectomy: a systematic review and evidence-based guidelines. Annals of Surgery. 2014 Mar;259(3):413–31. PubMed PMID: 24253135.

[186] Braga M, Ljungqvist O, Soeters P, Fearon K, Weimann A, Bozzetti F, et al. ESPEN Guidelines on parenteral nutrition: surgery. Clinical Nutrition. 2009 Aug;28(4):378–86. PubMed PMID: 19464088.

[187] Yang Z, Zheng Q, Wang Z. Meta-analysis of the need for nasogastric or nasojejunal decompression after gastrectomy for gastric cancer. British Journal of Surgery. 2008 Jul; 95(7):809–16. PubMed PMID: 18551533.

[188] Nelson R, Edwards S, Tse B. Prophylactic nasogastric decompression after abdominal surgery. Cochrane Database Systematic Reviews. 2007 (3):CD004929. PubMed PMID: 17636780.

[189] Sato T, Takayama T, So K, Murayama I. Is retention of a nasogastric tube after esophagectomy a risk factor for postoperative respiratory tract infection? Journal of Infection and Chemotherapy. 2007 Apr;13(2):109–13. PubMed PMID: 17458679.

[190] Shackcloth MJ, McCarron E, Kendall J, Russell GN, Pennefather SH, Tran J, et al. Randomized clinical trial to determine the effect of nasogastric drainage on tracheal acid aspiration following oesophagectomy. British Journal of Surgery. 2006 May;93(5): 547–52. PubMed PMID: 16521172.

[191] Suehiro T, Matsumata T, Shikada Y, Sugimachi K. Accelerated rehabilitation with early postoperative oral feeding following gastrectomy. Hepato-gastroenterology. 2004 Nov–Dec;51(60):1852–5. PubMed PMID: 15532842.

[192] Lassen K, Kjaeve J, Fetveit T, Trano G, Sigurdsson HK, Horn A, et al. Allowing normal food at will after major upper gastrointestinal surgery does not increase morbidity: a randomized multicenter trial. Annals of Surgery. 2008 May;247(5):721–9. PubMed PMID: 18438106.

[193] Convertino VA. Cardiovascular consequences of bed rest: effect on maximal oxygen uptake. Medicine & Science in Sports & Exercise. 1997 Feb;29(2):191–6. PubMed PMID: 9044222.

[194] Castelino T, Fiore JF, Jr., Niculiseanu P, Landry T, Augustin B, Feldman LS. The effect of early mobilization protocols on postoperative outcomes following abdominal and thoracic surgery: a systematic review. Surgery. 2016 Jan 21. PubMed PMID: 26804821.

http://dx.doi.org/10.5772/64775

[195] Aarts MA, Okrainec A, Glicksman A, Pearsall E, Victor JC, McLeod RS. Adoption of enhanced recovery after surgery (ERAS) strategies for colorectal surgery at academic teaching hospitals and impact on total length of hospital stay. Surgical Endoscopy. 2012 Feb;26(2):442–50. PubMed PMID: 22011937.

[196] Basse L, Raskov HH, Hjort Jakobsen D, Sonne E, Billesbolle P, Hendel HW, et al. Accelerated postoperative recovery programme after colonic resection improves physical performance, pulmonary function and body composition. The British Journal of Surgery. 2002 Apr;89(4):446–53. PubMed PMID: 11952586.

[197] Soreide E, Ljungqvist O. Modern preoperative fasting guidelines: a summary of the present recommendations and remaining questions. Best Practice & Research Clinical Anaesthesiology. 2006 Sep;20(3):483–91. PubMed PMID: 17080698.

[198] Mahajna A, Krausz M, Rosin D, Shabtai M, Hershko D, Ayalon A, et al. Bowel preparation is associated with spillage of bowel contents in colorectal surgery. Diseases of the Colon and Rectum. 2005 Aug;48(8):1626–31. PubMed PMID: 15981063.

[199] Englesbe MJ, Brooks L, Kubus J, Luchtefeld M, Lynch J, Senagore A, et al. A statewide assessment of surgical site infection following colectomy: the role of oral antibiotics. Annals of Surgery. 2010 Sep;252(3):514–9; discussion 9–20. PubMed PMID: 20739852. Pubmed Central PMCID: 2997819.

[200] Anthony T, Murray BW, Sum-Ping JT, Lenkovsky F, Vornik VD, Parker BJ, et al. Evaluating an evidence-based bundle for preventing surgical site infection: a randomized trial. Archives of Surgery. 2011 Mar;146(3):263–9. PubMed PMID: 21079110.

[201] Nelson RL, Gladman E, Barbateskovic M. Antimicrobial prophylaxis for colorectal surgery. The Cochrane Database of Systematic Reviews. 2014;5:CD001181. PubMed PMID: 24817514.

[202] Steinberg JP, Braun BI, Hellinger WC, Kusek L, Bozikis MR, Bush AJ, et al. Timing of antimicrobial prophylaxis and the risk of surgical site infections: results from the Trial to Reduce Antimicrobial Prophylaxis Errors. Annals of Surgery. 2009 Jul;250(1):10–16. PubMed PMID: 19561486.

[203] Jorgensen H, Wetterslev J, Moiniche S, Dahl JB. Epidural local anaesthetics versus opioid-based analgesic regimens on postoperative gastrointestinal paralysis, PONV and pain after abdominal surgery. The Cochrane Database of Systematic Reviews. 2000 (4):CD001893. PubMed PMID: 11034732.

[204] Marret E, Remy C, Bonnet F, Postoperative Pain Forum G. Meta-analysis of epidural analgesia versus parenteral opioid analgesia after colorectal surgery. The British Journal of Surgery. 2007 Jun;94(6):665–73. PubMed PMID: 17514701.

[205] Klein M. Postoperative non-steroidal anti-inflammatory drugs and colorectal anastomotic leakage. NSAIDs and anastomotic leakage. Dan Med J. 2012 Mar;59(3):B4420. PubMed PMID: 22381097. Epub 2012/03/03. eng.

[206] Gorissen KJ, Benning D, Berghmans T, Snoeijs MG, Sosef MN, Hulsewe KW, et al. Risk of anastomotic leakage with non-steroidal anti-inflammatory drugs in colorectal surgery. The British Journal of Surgery. 2012 May;99(5):721–7. PubMed PMID: 22318712. Epub 2012/02/10. eng.

[207] Klein M, Krarup PM, Burcharth J, Agren MS, Gogenur I, Jorgensen LN, et al. Effect of diclofenac on cyclooxygenase-2 levels and early breaking strength of experimental colonic anastomoses and skin incisions. European Surgical Research (Europaische chirurgische Forschung Recherches chirurgicales europeennes). 2011;46(1):26–31. PubMed PMID: 21135559. Epub 2010/12/08. eng.

[208] Hughes MJ, McNally S, Wigmore SJ. Enhanced recovery following liver surgery: a systematic review and meta-analysis. HPB (Oxford). 2014 Aug;16(8):699–706. PubMed PMID: 24661306. Pubmed Central PMCID: PMC4113251. Epub 2014/03/26. eng.

[209] Savikko J, Ilmakunnas M, Makisalo H, Nordin A, Isoniemi H. Enhanced recovery protocol after liver resection. British Journal of Surgery. 2015 Nov;102(12):1526–32. PubMed PMID: 26331595.

[210] van Dam RM, Wong-Lun-Hing EM, van Breukelen GJ, Stoot JH, van der Vorst JR, Bemelmans MH, et al. Open versus laparoscopic left lateral hepatic sectionectomy within an enhanced recovery ERAS(R) programme (ORANGE II-trial): study protocol for a randomised controlled trial. Trials. 2012;13:54. PubMed PMID: 22559239. Pubmed Central PMCID: 3409025.

[211] Mirnezami R, Mirnezami AH, Chandrakumaran K, Abu Hilal M, Pearce NW, Primrose JN, et al. Short- and long-term outcomes after laparoscopic and open hepatic resection: systematic review and meta-analysis. HPB (Oxford). 2011 May;13(5):295–308. PubMed PMID: 21492329. Pubmed Central PMCID: PMC3093641.

[212] Schiffman SC, Kim KH, Tsung A, Marsh JW, Geller DA. Laparoscopic versus open liver resection for metastatic colorectal cancer: a metaanalysis of 610 patients. Surgery. 2015 Feb;157(2):211–22. PubMed PMID: 25282529.

[213] Gurusamy KS, Samraj K, Davidson BR. Routine abdominal drainage for uncomplicated liver resection. Cochrane Database Systematic Reviews. 2007(3):CD006232. PubMed PMID: 17636837. Epub 2007/07/20. eng.

[214] Breitenstein S, DeOliveira ML, Raptis DA, Slankamenac K, Kambakamba P, Nerl J, et al. Novel and simple preoperative score predicting complications after liver resection in noncirrhotic patients. Annals of Surgery. 2010 Nov;252(5):726–34. PubMed PMID: 21037427.

[215] Zimmitti G, Roses RE, Andreou A, Shindoh J, Curley SA, Aloia TA, et al. Greater complexity of liver surgery is not associated with an increased incidence of liver-related complications except for bile leak: an experience with 2,628 consecutive resections. Journal of Gastrointestinal Surgery 2013 Jan;17(1):57–64; discussion p -5. PubMed PMID: 22956403. Pubmed Central PMCID: 3855461.

[216] Goonetilleke KS, Siriwardena AK. Systematic review of peri-operative nutritional supplementation in patients undergoing pancreaticoduodenectomy. JOP. 2006;7(1):5–13. PubMed PMID: 16407613.

[217] van der Gaag NA, Rauws EA, van Eijck CH, Bruno MJ, van der Harst E, Kubben FJ, et al. Preoperative biliary drainage for cancer of the head of the pancreas. New England Journal of Medicine. 2010 Jan 14;362(2):129–37. PubMed PMID: 20071702.

[218] Conlon KC, Labow D, Leung D, Smith A, Jarnagin W, Coit DG, et al. Prospective randomized clinical trial of the value of intraperitoneal drainage after pancreatic resection. Annals of Surgery. 2001 Oct;234(4):487–93; discussion 93–4. PubMed PMID: 11573042. Pubmed Central PMCID: 1422072.

[219] Bassi C, Molinari E, Malleo G, Crippa S, Butturini G, Salvia R, et al. Early versus late drain removal after standard pancreatic resections: results of a prospective randomized trial. Annals of Surgery. 2010 Aug;252(2):207–14. PubMed PMID: 20622661.

[220] Van Buren G, 2nd, Bloomston M, Hughes SJ, Winter J, Behrman SW, Zyromski NJ, et al. A randomized prospective multicenter trial of pancreaticoduodenectomy with and without routine intraperitoneal drainage. Annals of Surgery. 2014 Apr;259(4):605–12. PubMed PMID: 24374513.

[221] Wang YC, Szatmary P, Zhu JQ, Xiong JJ, Huang W, Gomatos I, et al. Prophylactic intra-peritoneal drain placement following pancreaticoduodenectomy: a systematic review and meta-analysis. World Journal of Gastroenterology. 2015 Feb 28;21(8):2510–21. PubMed PMID: 25741162. Pubmed Central PMCID: PMC4342931.

[222] American Thoracic S, American College of Chest P. ATS/ACCP Statement on cardio-pulmonary exercise testing. American Journal of Respiratory and Critical Care Medicine. 2003 Jan 15;167(2):211–77. PubMed PMID: 12524257.

[223] Moran J, Wilson F, Guinan E, McCormick P, Hussey J, Moriarty J. Role of cardiopulmonary exercise testing as a risk-assessment method in patients undergoing intra-abdominal surgery: a systematic review. British Journal of Anaesthesia. 2016 Feb;116(2): 177–91. PubMed PMID: 26787788.

[224] Dunne DF, Jones RP, Lythgoe DT, Pilkington FJ, Palmer DH, Malik HZ, et al. Cardio-pulmonary exercise testing before liver surgery. Journal of Surgical Oncology. 2014 Sep; 110(4):439–44. PubMed PMID: 24894657. Epub 2014/06/05. eng.

[225] Ausania F, Snowden CP, Prentis JM, Holmes LR, Jaques BC, White SA, et al. Effects of low cardiopulmonary reserve on pancreatic leak following pancreaticoduodenectomy. British Journal of Surgery. 2012 Sep;99(9):1290–4. PubMed PMID: 22828960. Epub 2012/07/26. eng.

[226] Remels AH, Gosker HR, Schrauwen P, Langen RC, Schols AM. Peroxisome proliferator-activated receptors: a therapeutic target in COPD? The European Respiratory Journal. 2008 Mar;31(3):502–8. PubMed PMID: 18310397.

[227] Sandri M, Lin J, Handschin C, Yang W, Arany ZP, Lecker SH, et al. PGC-1alpha protects skeletal muscle from atrophy by suppressing FoxO3 action and atrophy-specific gene transcription. Proceedings of the National Academy of Sciences of the United States of America. 2006 Oct 31;103(44):16260–5. PubMed PMID: 17053067. Pubmed Central PMCID: 1637570.

[228] Mayo NE, Feldman L, Scott S, Zavorsky G, Kim do J, Charlebois P, et al. Impact of preoperative change in physical function on postoperative recovery: argument supporting prehabilitation for colorectal surgery. Surgery. 2011 Sep;150(3):505–14. PubMed PMID: 21878237.

[229] Dale W, Hemmerich J, Kamm A, Posner MC, Matthews JB, Rothman R, et al. Geriatric assessment improves prediction of surgical outcomes in older adults undergoing pancreaticoduodenectomy: a prospective cohort study. Annals of Surgery. 2014 May; 259(5):960–5. PubMed PMID: 24096757.

[230] Breen L, Phillips SM. Skeletal muscle protein metabolism in the elderly: interventions to counteract the 'anabolic resistance' of ageing. Nutrition & Metabolism. 2011;8:68. PubMed PMID: 21975196. Pubmed Central PMCID: 3201893.

[231] Volpi E, Kobayashi H, Sheffield-Moore M, Mittendorfer B, Wolfe RR. Essential amino acids are primarily responsible for the amino acid stimulation of muscle protein anabolism in healthy elderly adults. The American Journal of Clinical Nutrition. 2003 Aug;78(2):250–8. PubMed PMID: 12885705. Pubmed Central PMCID: 3192452.

[232] Kornasio R, Riederer I, Butler-Browne G, Mouly V, Uni Z, Halevy O. Beta-hydroxy-beta-methylbutyrate (HMB) stimulates myogenic cell proliferation, differentiation and survival via the MAPK/ERK and PI3K/Akt pathways. Biochimica et Biophysica Acta. 2009 May;1793(5):755–63. PubMed PMID: 19211028.

[233] Vukovich MD, Stubbs NB, Bohlken RM. Body composition in 70-year-old adults responds to dietary beta-hydroxy-beta-methylbutyrate similarly to that of young adults. The Journal of Nutrition. 2001 Jul;131(7):2049–52. PubMed PMID: 11435528.

[234] Flakoll P, Sharp R, Baier S, Levenhagen D, Carr C, Nissen S. Effect of beta-hydroxy-beta-methylbutyrate, arginine, and lysine supplementation on strength, functionality, body composition, and protein metabolism in elderly women. Nutrition. 2004 May; 20(5):445–51. PubMed PMID: 15105032.

[235] Baier S, Johannsen D, Abumrad N, Rathmacher JA, Nissen S, Flakoll P. Year-long changes in protein metabolism in elderly men and women supplemented with a nutrition cocktail of beta-hydroxy-beta-methylbutyrate (HMB), L-arginine, and L-lysine. JPEN Journal of Parenteral and Enteral Nutrition. 2009 Jan–Feb;33(1):71–82. PubMed PMID: 19164608.

[236] Li C, Carli F, Lee L, Charlebois P, Stein B, Liberman AS, et al. Impact of a trimodal prehabilitation program on functional recovery after colorectal cancer surgery: a pilot study. Surgical Endoscopy. 2013 Apr;27(4):1072–82. PubMed PMID: 23052535.

[237] van Waart H, Stuiver MM, van Harten WH, Geleijn E, Kieffer JM, Buffart LM, et al. Effect of low-intensity physical activity and moderate- to high-intensity physical exercise during adjuvant chemotherapy on physical fitness, fatigue, and chemotherapy completion rates: results of the PACES Randomized Clinical Trial. Journal of Clinical Oncology: Official Journal of the American Society of Clinical Oncology. 2015 Jun 10;33(17):1918–27. PubMed PMID: 25918291.

[238] Smets EM, Garssen B, Bonke B, De Haes JC. The Multidimensional Fatigue Inventory (MFI) psychometric qualities of an instrument to assess fatigue. Journal of Psychosomatic Research. 1995 Apr;39(3):315–25. PubMed PMID: 7636775.

[239] Gielissen MF, Verhagen S, Witjes F, Bleijenberg G. Effects of cognitive behavior therapy in severely fatigued disease-free cancer patients compared with patients waiting for cognitive behavior therapy: a randomized controlled trial. Journal of Clinical Oncology: Official Journal of the American Society of Clinical Oncology. 2006 Oct 20;24(30):4882–7. PubMed PMID: 17050873.

[240] Goedendorp MM, Gielissen MF, Verhagen CA, Bleijenberg G. Psychosocial interventions for reducing fatigue during cancer treatment in adults. The Cochrane Database of Systematic Reviews. 2009;(1):CD006953. PubMed PMID: 19160308.

[241] Nitenberg G, Raynard B. Nutritional support of the cancer patient: issues and dilemmas. Critical Reviews in Oncology/Hematology. 2000 Jun;34(3):137–68. PubMed PMID: 10838261.

[242] Garth AK, Newsome CM, Simmance N, Crowe TC. Nutritional status, nutrition practices and post-operative complications in patients with gastrointestinal cancer. Journal of Human Nutrition and Dietetics: The Official Journal of the British Dietetic Association. 2010 Aug;23(4):393–401. PubMed PMID: 20337847.

[243] Afaneh C, Gerszberg D, Slattery E, Seres DS, Chabot JA, Kluger MD. Pancreatic cancer surgery and nutrition management: a review of the current literature. Hepatobiliary Surgery and Nutrition. 2015 Feb;4(1):59–71. PubMed PMID: 25713805. Pubmed Central PMCID: 4318958.

[244] Schindler K, Pernicka E, Laviano A, Howard P, Schutz T, Bauer P, et al. How nutritional risk is assessed and managed in European hospitals: a survey of 21,007 patients findings from the 2007–2008 cross-sectional nutritionDay survey. Clinical Nutrition. 2010 Oct; 29(5):552–9. PubMed PMID: 20434820.

[245] Skipworth RJ, Fearon KC. The scientific rationale for optimizing nutritional support in cancer. European Journal of Gastroenterology & Hepatology. 2007 May;19(5):371–7. PubMed PMID: 17413286.

[246] Loh KW, Vriens MR, Gerritsen A, Borel Rinkes IH, van Hillegersberg R, Schippers C, et al. Unintentional weight loss is the most important indicator of malnutrition among surgical cancer patients. The Netherlands Journal of Medicine. 2012 Oct;70(8):365–9. PubMed PMID: 23065984.

[247] Martin L, Senesse P, Gioulbasanis I, Antoun S, Bozzetti F, Deans C, et al. Diagnostic criteria for the classification of cancer-associated weight loss. Journal of Clinical Oncology: Official Journal of the American Society of Clinical Oncology. 2015 Jan 1;33(1):90–9. PubMed PMID: 25422490.

[248] Gonzalez MC, Pastore CA, Orlandi SP, Heymsfield SB. Obesity paradox in cancer: new insights provided by body composition. The American Journal of Clinical Nutrition. 2014 May;99(5):999–1005. PubMed PMID: 24572565.

Chapter 4

Infections in Cancer Patients

Deepjot Singh and Robert A. Bonomo

Additional information is available at the end of the chapter

http://dx.doi.org/10.5772/64372

Abstract

Cancer therapy is a dynamically evolving field. Chemotherapy and biologic agents impact the magnitude and duration of immunosuppression in the already-immunocompromised cancer hosts who are then susceptible to a broad spectrum of infectious complications ranging from mild opportunistic infections to severe, fatal neutropenic sepsis. Numerous bacterial, fungal, and viral organisms have been implicated dictating varied preventative approaches. Rapid assessment and risk stratification of febrile patients identify individuals requiring hospital admission. Timely delivery of antimicrobials reduces the risk of complications and death. Herein, we summarize the current "state of art" in the management of infection in the cancer patient. We detail the advances in antibacterial and antifungal therapy.

Keywords: Cancer, Fever, Infection, Neutropenia, Chemotherapy

1. Introduction

Cancer patients are at a risk for development of severe infections. Predisposing factors include severe neutropenia, impaired neutrophil function, and B-cell, T-cell, or NK-cell defects. Patients with chronic lymphocytic leukemia often have hypogammaglobulinemia which increases susceptibility to encapsulated bacteria. Patients with advanced solid tumors including head and neck cancer, lung cancer, gastrointestinal malignancy, and pancreatic cancer are commonly malnourished. Malnutrition impairs immune function and increases the susceptibility to infection. Chemotherapy, biological agents, and high-dose steroids may also cause significant immunosuppression, thereby increasing the risk for infection. In the United States, approximately 60,000 patients are admitted due to neutropenia, annually. One in fourteen of these patients dies secondary to sepsis-related complications [1]. The estimated daily cost of hospitalization is $2,000–$3,000 [2]. Advances in infection control and antimicrobial stewardship are therefore important to diminish the impact of infections in these immunocompromised hosts.

2. Cancer therapy–related infections

Most single chemotherapeutic agents used for the treatment of solid tumors do not cause prolonged neutropenia and are therefore associated with a low risk for bacterial infections. Additionally, they do not cause significant suppression of T-cell function leading to clinically relevant viral reactivation. On the other hand, induction and consolidation chemotherapy for acute leukemia may result in severe, prolonged neutropenia, thereby not only increasing the risk of bacterial and fungal infections but also predisposing to herpes simplex virus (HSV) reactivation [3].

Epidermal growth factor receptor (EGFR) inhibitors are commonly used in the treatment of solid tumors. Cetuximab is a chimeric murine-human IgG1 monoclonal antibody that is used in the treatment of head and neck cancer and advanced colorectal cancer. Panitumumab is a fully human IgG2 monoclonal antibody used in the treatment of advanced colorectal cancer. Erlotinib and gefitinib are used in the treatment of lung adenocarcinoma. These EGFR inhibitors may be associated with acneiform eruptions and paronychia. Severe skin toxicities complicated by infection, abscess, and sepsis have also been reported. Trastuzumab and pertuzumab are anti-HER2 monoclonal antibodies used in the treatment of breast cancer. In a meta-analysis of 13 randomized studies of breast cancer patients ($N = 10{,}094$), treatment with trastuzumab was associated with 8.5 % (95 % CI 4.5–15.4 %) incidence of high-grade infection and 12.0 % (95 % CI 8.1–17.4 %) incidence of febrile neutropenia in the absence of high-grade neutropenia or leukopenia [4].

Mammalian target of rapamycin (mTOR) inhibitors (temsirolimus and everolimus) is used in the treatment of advanced renal cell carcinoma. Severe lymphopenia, neutropenia, and sepsis have been reported. Immunosuppression with these agents may increase the risk of opportunistic infections including *Pneumocystis jiroveci* pneumonia (PJP). In a meta-analysis of ten randomized trials of cancer patients ($N = 3{,}535$), everolimus and temsirolimus were associated with a 21 % (95 % CI 15.0–28.9 %) risk of high-grade infections [5].

Vascular endothelial growth factor receptor/tyrosine kinase inhibitors (VEGFR-TKIs) block angiogenesis by inhibiting VEGF and other growth factors. They are used in the treatment of a variety of tumors including chronic myelogenous leukemia (imatinib, dasatinib, nilotinib), renal cancer (sunitinib, sorafenib, pazopanib, and axitinib), hepatocellular carcinoma (sorafenib), colorectal cancer (regorafenib), thyroid cancer (sorafenib, vandetanib), and sarcoma (cediranib). In a meta-analysis of 27 randomized trials ($N = 16{,}488$), VEGFR-TKIs significantly increased the risk of developing severe (1.69-fold) and fatal infectious events (1.78-fold) in cancer patients [6].

Monoclonal antibodies that target B lymphocytes cause significant cellular immunosuppression predisposing to bacterial, fungal, and viral infections. Reactivation of hepatitis B virus (HBV) is more common compared to other viruses such as herpes simplex virus (HSV), varicella zoster virus (VZV), cytomegalovirus (CMV), and Epstein-Barr virus (EBV) [7]. These agents should not be administered to patients with active infection. Anti-CD20-directed monoclonal antibodies (rituximab, ofatumumab, and obinutuzumab) are used in the treatment of lymphoproliferative disorders. Their use is associated with HBV reactivation resulting in fulminant hepatitis, hepatic failure, and death [8, 9]. Anti-CD30-directed monoclonal antibody (brentuximab vedotin) is used in the management of relapsed Hodgkin's lymphoma and anaplastic large-cell lymphoma. Its use is associated with prolonged severe neutropenia and neutropenic fever. Cases of progressive multifocal leukoencephalopathy (PML) and death due to JC virus infection have also been reported [10]. Anti-CD38-directed monoclonal antibody (daratumumab) is used in the management of refractory multiple myeloma. Its use is associated with myelosuppression. Herpes zoster occurs in 3 % of patients. Antiviral prophylaxis to prevent herpes zoster reactivation should be initiated within one week of starting daratumumab and continued for three months following the last dose [11]. Anti-CD52-directed monoclonal antibody (alemtuzumab) is used for treatment of chronic lymphocytic leukemia. It induces severe and prolonged lymphopenia and increases the risk of serious and potentially fatal bacterial, viral, fungal, and protozoan infections. Prophylactic medications against PJP and herpes virus infection during treatment and for at least 2 months following last dose or until CD4+ counts are ≥200 cells/μL are recommended. Close monitoring for CMV reactivation is also recommended [12].

Signaling lymphocyte activation molecule family 7 (SLAMF7) is present on myeloma cells and natural killer cells. Anti-SLAMF7-directed monoclonal antibody (elotuzumab) is administered in combination with lenalidomide and dexamethasone for refractory myeloma. Bone marrow suppression and increased risk of opportunistic, fungal, and herpes zoster infection have been reported [13].

Janus kinase (JAK) 1/2 inhibitor, ruxolitinib, is used for the treatment of polycythemia vera and myelofibrosis. Its use is associated with impairment of dendritic cell and T-cell function and reduction in cytokines resulting in the development of serious bacterial, fungal, and viral infections. Opportunistic infections reported include HBV reactivation, disseminated tuberculosis, *Cryptococcus* pneumonia, toxoplasmosis retinitis, and PML [14, 15].

Checkpoint inhibitors target cytotoxic T-lymphocyte-associated antigen 4 (CTLA-4) and programmed cell death-1 (PD-1) receptor. Anti-CTLA-4 antibody (ipilimumab) is used in the treatment of melanoma. Anti-PD-1 antibodies (nivolumab and pembrolizumab) are used in the management of melanoma and lung cancer. Checkpoint inhibition is associated with immune-mediated adverse events including pneumonitis, colitis, hepatitis, nephritis, dermatitis, and endocrinopathies. High-dose glucocorticoids are used in the management of grade 2 or greater immune-related toxicities, which increase the risk for development of opportunistic infections.

3. Role of antimicrobial prophylaxis in the prevention of cancer-related infections

Infection risk in patients with cancer depends on several factors including age more than 65 years, tumor burden (size and number of lesions), regimen and intensity of cytotoxic chemotherapy, duration of neutropenia, degree of mucositis, and associated comorbidities. Intense cytotoxic chemotherapy causes prolonged neutropenia which impairs the inflammatory response and predisposes the individual to serious infection(**Figure 1**).

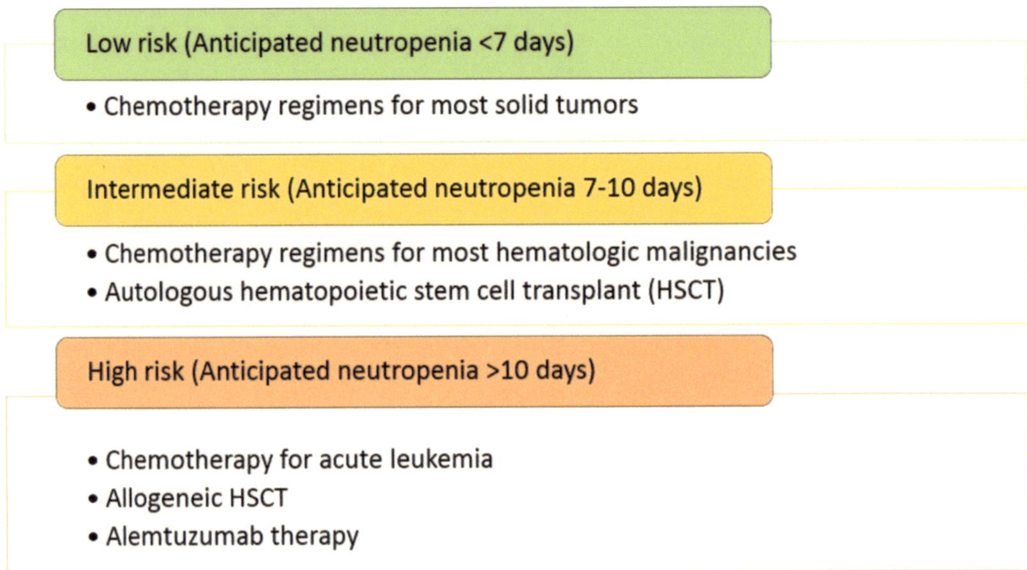

Figure 1. National Comprehensive Cancer Network (NCCN) criteria for risk of infection in patients undergoing chemotherapy [16].

Neutropenia is a major risk factor for the development of infections. Neutropenic fever is more common after chemotherapy for hematologic malignancies than solid tumors. Preventive measures against infections involve antimicrobial prophylaxis for patients receiving chemotherapy regimens associated with greater than or equal to twenty percent risk for fever and neutropenia.

3.1. Antibacterial prophylaxis during neutropenia

Patients receiving combination or dose-intensive chemotherapy are at increased risk for prolonged neutropenia [absolute neutrophil count (ANC) $< 1,000/\mu L$ lasting more than 7 days] and bacterial infections. Gram-negative bacilli are associated with life-threatening infections. In a meta-analysis of neutropenic patients (18 trials, $N = 1,408$) with solid tumors and hematological malignancies, fluoroquinolone prophylaxis (ciprofloxacin, norfloxacin, enoxacin, and ofloxacin) significantly lowered the incidence of gram-negative infections by 80 % (RR, 0.21; 95 % CI 0.12–0.37) when compared with placebo and by 70 % when compared with trimethoprim-sulfamethoxazole (TMP-SMX). Quinolone prophylaxis did not alter the incidence of gram-positive bacterial and fungal infections or infection-related deaths [17]. In another meta-analysis of afebrile neutropenic patients (109 trials, *N* = 13,579) with hematologic malignancies, antibiotic prophylaxis significantly decreased all-cause mortality (RR 0.66, 95 % CI 0.55–0.79) and infection-related mortality (RR 0.61, 95 % CI 0.48–0.77) compared to placebo or no intervention. Quinolone prophylaxis was associated with the most significant reduction in mortality [18]. Ciprofloxacin is more potent than levofloxacin against gram-negative bacteria. Nevertheless, levofloxacin with wider activity against gram-positive cocci may benefit as a prophylactic agent for mucositis-associated infections.

Levofloxacin prophylaxis in high-risk patients with anticipated prolonged neutropenia reduces clinically significant bacterial infections including gram-negative bacteremia [19]. Prophylaxis in low-risk patients with anticipated short-duration neutropenia decreases fever and hospitalization for febrile neutropenia, but not infection-related mortality [20]. Fluoroquinolone use may be associated with hypersensitivity reactions, prolonged QTc interval, tendon rupture, peripheral neuropathy, seizures, *Clostridium difficile* diarrhea, *Streptococcus viridans* bacteremia, and methicillin-resistant *Staphylococcus aureus* (MRSA) infection [21–23].

The National Comprehensive Cancer Network (NCCN) guidelines panel recommends the use of fluoroquinolone prophylaxis (levofloxacin) for patients with anticipated prolonged neutropenia. Antibacterial prophylaxis is not recommended for anticipated short-duration neutropenia due to the risk of emergence of quinolone-resistant bacteria [24].

3.2. Antifungal prophylaxis

Patients with acute myeloid leukemia (AML) and myelodysplastic syndrome (MDS) and allogeneic hematopoietic stem cell transplant (HSCT) recipients are at increased risk for life-threatening infections with yeasts or molds. *Candida* and *Aspergillus* species are the most common pathogens. Amphotericin B (AMB) has activity against both *Candida* spp. and *Aspergillus* spp. but is too toxic for antifungal prophylaxis.

Studies supporting antifungal prophylaxis in patients undergoing induction chemotherapy for AML have shown that fluconazole is superior to placebo in preventing invasive candidiasis [25] and is as effective as amphotericin B [26]. However, fluconazole lacks activity against molds. Itraconazole has activity against both *Candida* and *Aspergillus* species. It significantly reduces invasive fungal disease (IFD) compared to fluconazole at the cost of greater toxicity [27–29]. Voriconazole is active against a wider range of fungi including *Candida* spp., *Aspergillus* spp., *Scedosporium* spp., and *Fusarium* spp. [30]. Nevertheless, data supporting voriconazole prophylaxis in the non-transplant AML population is limited. Posaconazole has broader antifungal coverage including *Candida* spp., *Aspergillus* spp., *Scedosporium* spp., *Fusarium* spp., and *Mucorales*. It is the only agent that has demonstrated survival benefit in prophylaxis against mycosis during AML induction therapy [31]. Azoles (itraconazole, voriconazole, and posaconazole) inhibit cytochrome P450 3A4 isoenzyme and may decrease the clearance of antineoplastic agent vincristine. Caspofungin is active against both *Candida* and *Aspergillus* spp. It has similar efficacy as itraconazole and is better tolerated [32]. It may therefore be a reasonable substitute for antifungal prophylaxis in patients who are unable to tolerate oral posaconazole.

Antifungal prophylaxis in patients undergoing HSCT is more complex due to concerns for poor oral absorption due to mucositis and drug interactions with antineoplastic and immunosuppressive medications. Fluconazole decreases invasive candidiasis and IFD-related mortality. Itraconazole has superior efficacy than fluconazole in prevention of IFD. Coadministration of itraconazole with antineoplastic conditioning regimens containing cyclophosphamide is associated with increased incidence of renal and hepatic toxicities. Voriconazole is as effective as itraconazole and is better tolerated [33]. Micafungin is as efficacious as itraconazole with less toxicity [34]. In patients with GVHD requiring immunosuppressive therapy, posaconazole has demonstrated improvement in IFD-related mortality (1 % vs. 4 %, $p = .046$) compared to fluconazole [35, 36] (**Figure 2**).

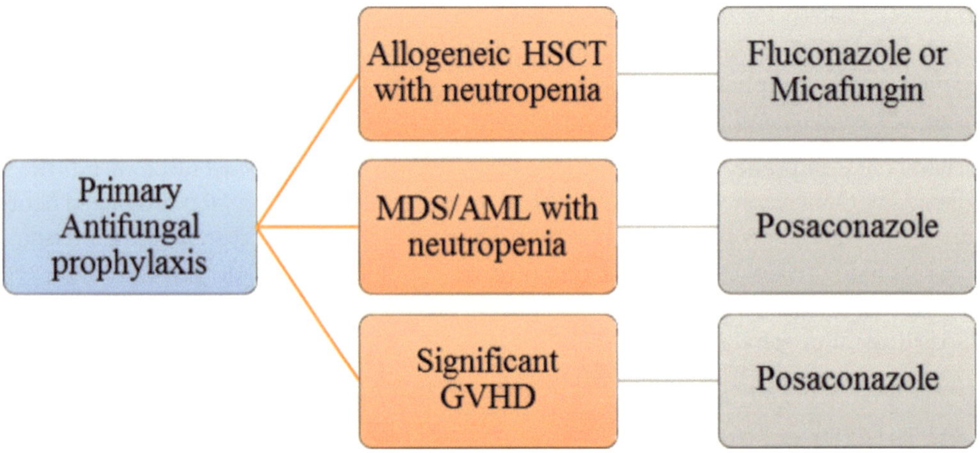

Figure 2. Primary antifungal prophylaxis in patients with hematologic disorders. HSCT, hematopoietic stem cell transplant; MDS, myelodysplastic syndrome; AML, acute myeloid leukemia; GVHD, graft-versus-host disease.

3.3. Anti-pneumocystis prophylaxis

P. jiroveci pneumonia (PJP) is a potentially life-threatening infection that may occur in immunocompromised individuals with acute lymphocytic leukemia (ALL) and recipients of allogeneic HSCT and alemtuzumab therapy. Patients receiving purine analog therapy, temozolomide in conjunction with radiation therapy, and high-dose glucocorticoids (equivalent to ≥20 mg of prednisone daily for 4 or more weeks) may also be at risk.

In patients with AML or solid organ transplantation, prophylaxis with TMP/SMX compared to no treatment or treatment with fluoroquinolones reduced the incidence of PJP infections by 85 % (RR 0.15, 95 % CI 0.04–0.62; ten trials, 1,000 patients) and PJP-related mortality by 83 % (RR 0.17, 95 % CI 0.03–0.94; nine trials, 886 patients). Reduction in all-cause mortality was not observed. There was also no difference between once daily vs. thrice weekly TMP/SMX [37].

TMP/SMX is superior to dapsone and pentamidine in allogeneic HSCT recipients [38, 39]. PJP prophylaxis is administered for six months in allogeneic HSCT recipients and longer in patients with GVHD. ALL patients should receive prophylaxis till completion of immunosuppressive therapy. For those receiving alemtuzumab, anti-PJP prophylaxis is continued for a minimum of 2 months beyond alemtuzumab therapy or when the CD4+ cell count is above 200 cells/μL [16].

3.4. Antiviral prophylaxis

Most cancer patients are at low risk of contracting viral infections. Immunosuppression may however predispose them to respiratory tract viral infections. Reactivation of HSV, VZV, and HBV is more likely to occur during intensive chemotherapy. EBV and CMV occur in the setting of allogeneic HSCT. The risk of viral infection increases with the intensity and duration of T-cell suppression. The extent of neutropenia is less important.

3.4.1. Influenza virus

Inactivated influenza vaccine is administered annually to patients undergoing chemotherapy [40]. Patients receiving induction or consolidation therapy for AML or those who have received anti-B-cell antibody within the last six months are excluded. Vaccination should be administered at least two weeks prior to receiving immunosuppressive therapy. Patients should be considered unprotected if they were vaccinated less than 2 weeks before start of immunosuppressive therapy. These patients should be revaccinated at least three months after the cytotoxic therapy is discontinued [41]. Acute leukemics should be vaccinated after completion of chemotherapy. Patients with ALL should receive the vaccine during the maintenance phase of their therapy [42].

3.4.2. Hepatitis B virus (HBV)

Reactivation of latent HBV occurs in patients with leukemia (ALL, AML, and chronic lymphocytic leukemia (CLL)), lymphoma, myeloma, and breast cancer, transplant recipients, or patients receiving high-dose steroids, anti-CD 20 antibodies, alemtuzumab, or purine analogs. Screening tests include hepatitis B surface antigen (HBsAg), hepatitis B core antibody (anti-HBc), and HBV DNA. Patients who are HBsAg positive/anti-HBc positive or HBsAg negative/anti-HBc positive are at risk for reactivation. Antiviral therapy should be initiated in patients with HBsAg-positive/anti-HBc-positive serology either prior to or concurrent with cytotoxic therapy. HBsAg-negative/anti-HBc-positive patients may be monitored for reactivation with HBV DNA and Alanine Transferase (ALT) levels and antivirals initiated at reactivation. Evidence of reactivation includes change in the HBV DNA from undetectable to detectable, or ≥1 log rise in HBV DNA level above baseline, or seroconversion from negative to positive HBsAg status. ALT should be monitored to assess hepatic function in the setting of HBV reactivation [43]. HBV DNA is monitored monthly during cytotoxic therapy and then every 3 months after completion of therapy. Antiviral therapy should be continued for 6 months after completion of cytotoxic therapy and for longer than 12 months in patients treated with anti-CD 20 monoclonal antibodies. HBV prophylaxis results in 87 % relative risk reduction of reactivation [43]. It also prevents fulminant hepatitis [44]. Entecavir is more effective than lamivudine and is associated with lower incidence of viral resistance and hepatitis [9]. Allogeneic HSCT candidates with evidence of active HBV infection should receive antiviral therapy for three to six months prior to initiation of conditioning [45].

3.4.3. Herpes simplex virus (HSV)

Reactivation and infection with HSV occur in patients undergoing induction therapy for acute leukemia and HSCT recipients. Prolonged neutropenia and mucositis are major predisposing factors. The risk of HSV reactivation is highest in the first 30 days following allogeneic transplant. Screening tests include HSV-1 and HSV-2 IgG antibodies. In a meta-analysis of nine randomized trials of HSCT recipients, acyclovir prophylaxis reduced HSV infection (RR 0.19, 95 % CI 0.11–0.31) without impacting overall mortality [46]. Antiviral prophylaxis with *acyclovir* or *valacyclovir* is therefore recommended in HSV-seropositive patients. The antiviral agent is administered with the initiation of the conditioning regimen and is continued till either engraftment occurs or the mucositis has resolved. Patients with chronic lymphocytic leukemia (CLL) receiving alemtuzumab therapy are also at risk for HSV infection. Antiviral prophylaxis is recommended for 2 months beyond alemtuzumab therapy or when the CD4+ cell count is above 200 cells/μL [47].

3.4.4. Varicella zoster virus (VZV)

Reactivation of VZV occurs in seropositive HSCT recipients. Screening test includes VZV IgG antibody. Antiviral prophylaxis with acyclovir or valacyclovir for one year post transplant significantly reduces reactivation compared to no therapy (9 % vs. 25 %, $p < 0.001$) [48]. Patients receiving T-cell-depleting agents (proteasome inhibitors, purine analogs, and prednisone ≥ 1 mg/kg/day) are also at risk for VZV infection. Antiviral prophylaxis is continued until the immunosuppressive therapy is completed [49]. Recommendations for CLL patients receiving alemtuzumab include continuing VZV prophylaxis for 2 months beyond completion of treatment or when the CD4+ cell count is above 200 cells/μL.

3.4.5. Cytomegalovirus (CMV)

Reactivation and infection with CMV occur in allogeneic hematopoietic transplant recipients and patients receiving alemtuzumab treatment [50]. Screening test includes weekly quantitative CMV testing (CMV DNA by polymerase chain reaction (PCR) or CMV pp65 antigen from peripheral blood leukocytes). CMV blood testing is done for at least six months after allogeneic HSCT. Patient receiving alemtuzumab therapy should undergo surveillance during treatment and for at least 2 months after completion of treatment. Preemptive therapy for patients with CMV viremia is recommended rather than administering toxic antiviral prophylaxis. Treatment is continued for 2 weeks or until CMV viremia is no longer detectable. First-line therapy includes intravenous ganciclovir or oral valganciclovir. Ganciclovir is associated with bone marrow suppression. Second-line option foscarnet is nephrotoxic. Both acyclovir and valacyclovir are less toxic and also less active than ganciclovir.

http://dx.doi.org/10.5772/64372

4. Management of febrile neutropenia

4.1. Definitions

Fever is defined as a single oral temperature of ≥38.3 °C (101 °F) or a temperature of ≥38.0 °C (100.4 °F) for 1 h or longer [24]. Neutropenia is defined as an absolute neutrophil count (ANC) of <1,000 cells/μL. Severe neutropenia is defined as an ANC of <500 cells/μL. Profound neutropenia is defined as an ANC of <100 cells/μL. Prolonged profound neutropenia (lasting >7 days) is likely to occur in patients undergoing induction chemotherapy for acute leukemia or after allogeneic HSCT. Functional neutropenia occurs in patients with hematologic malignancy whose circulating neutrophils have impaired phagocytosis. These patients are at risk of infection despite "normal" neutrophil counts [51].

4.2. Initial assessment and investigations

Febrile neutropenia is a medical emergency requiring immediate evaluation and administration of empiric broad-spectrum antibiotics within an hour of presentation [24]. The initial assessment focuses on not only determining the probable site of infection but also the patient's risk of developing serious complications and the need for vigorous resuscitation. Relevant historical information should include the chemotherapy regimen, number of chemotherapy cycles, days since receiving anticancer treatment, concomitant use of biologic agents and steroids, growth factor support, prophylactic antimicrobials, recent surgery or radiation therapy, prior infections, HIV status, and other comorbid illnesses. Laboratory evaluation should include complete blood count with differential, renal, and hepatic function tests and cultures from all potential sites including sputum, urine, stool, skin, and mucosal ulcers as clinically relevant. At least two sets of blood cultures from peripheral veins or one set each from a peripheral vein and a central venous catheter should be drawn. Chest radiographs should be evaluated in patients with signs or symptoms of lower respiratory tract infection.

4.3. Risk stratification

Patients with febrile neutropenia are risk stratified into high- or low-risk groups based on the probability of development of serious infection-related complications.

4.3.1. The Talcott model

Patients are assigned to one of four Talcott model risk groups in the first 24 h of presentation. In the prospective validation study of this model ($N = 444$), medical complications developed in 5 % group IV patients compared to 34 % in combined groups I–III ($p < .000001$). There were no deaths in group IV patients compared to 10 % deaths in combined groups I–III. Medical complications included hypotension, tachyarrhythmias, congestive heart failure, respiratory failure, serious bleeding, altered mental status, new focal neurologic changes, and intensive care admission [52] (**Figure 3**).

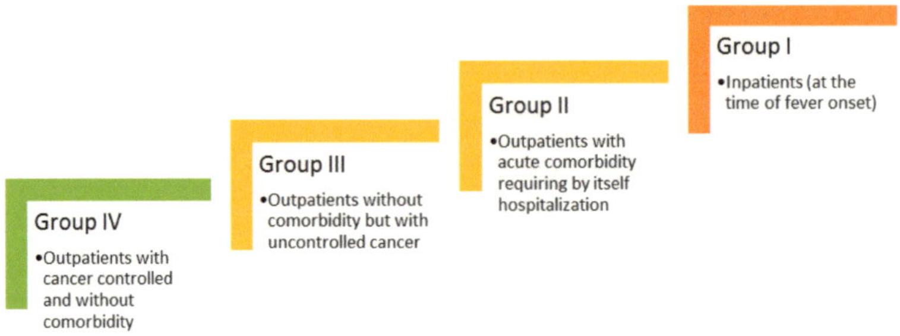

Figure 3. The Talcott model.

4.3.2. The MASCC risk index

The Multinational Association for Supportive Care in Cancer (MASCC) risk index uses weighted scores based on disease burden, clinical instability, age, and comorbid conditions.

The maximum theoretical MASCC score is 26. Low-risk patients have a MASCC score ≥21 and mortality as low as 3 %. High-risk patients with MASCC score <15 have a mortality as high as 36 %. The MASCC rule does not consider the duration of anticipated neutropenia as a criteria for risk stratification [53]. Both Talcott model and MASCC index score are used to identify low-risk febrile neutropenic patients who are suitable for outpatient management.

4.3.3. The NCCN model [16]

The NCCN guidelines panel considers high-risk febrile neutropenic patients as those with MASCC scores of less than 21. The panel further recommends that patients with prolonged profound neutropenia should be considered high risk, regardless of the MASCC risk index score. Other factors stratifying patients as high risk include those noted in **Figure 4**. These high-risk febrile neutropenic patients require hospital admission and parenteral therapy (**Figure 5**).

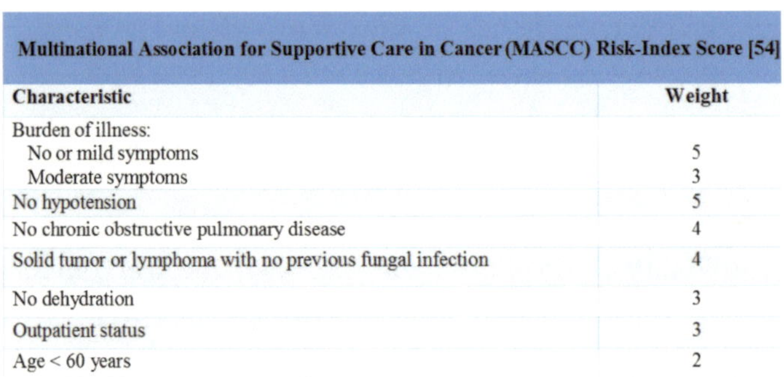

Multinational Association for Supportive Care in Cancer (MASCC) Risk-Index Score [54]	
Characteristic	**Weight**
Burden of illness:	
No or mild symptoms	5
Moderate symptoms	3
No hypotension	5
No chronic obstructive pulmonary disease	4
Solid tumor or lymphoma with no previous fungal infection	4
No dehydration	3
Outpatient status	3
Age < 60 years	2

Figure 4. The MASCC risk index score.

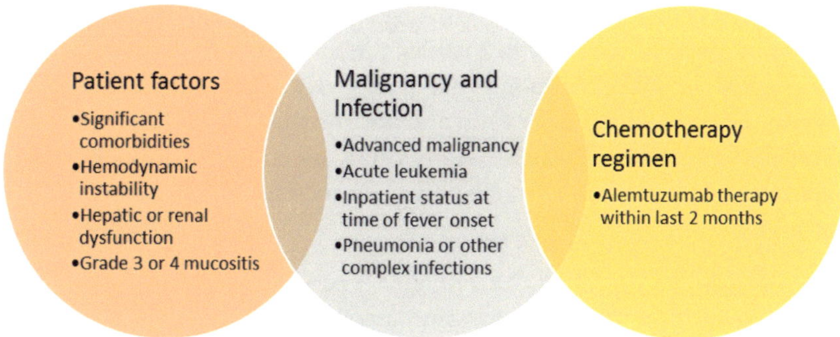

Figure 5. High-risk factors in febrile neutropenic patients.

4.4. Outpatient therapy for low-risk patients

Febrile neutropenic patients with MASCC scores ≥ 21 or in Talcott group 4 are at low risk for infection-related complications provided they do not have active comorbidities or organ dysfunction. These patients can be managed safely as outpatients if they live close to a medical facility, agree to frequent clinic visits, and have 24-h caregiver support at home with easy access to telephone and transportation. Low-risk patients should receive initial doses of empirical antibacterial therapy within an hour of triage. They should then undergo a brief period of observation (at least 4 h) in a medical facility to determine the suitability for outpatient management or the need for hospitalization [51].

The majority of febrile neutropenic episodes in patients receiving chemotherapy for solid tumors are low risk. Bacterial infections are the presumed culprits for unexplained fever. Fungal infections are uncommon, and reactivation of viruses is rare. In a cohort of low-risk febrile neutropenic patients ($N = 757$), unexplained febrile episodes were predominant (58 %), followed by equal frequency (21 %) of both clinically significant and microbiologically documented infections. The most common clinical sites of infection were the upper respiratory tract and skin. Among microbiologically documented infections, monomicrobial gram-positive infections accounted for 49 % (coagulase-negative staphylococci most frequent) followed by monomicrobial gram-negative infections (36 %, *Escherichia coli* predominant) and polymicrobial infections (15 %) [54].

Two randomized control trials (RCTs) of low-risk febrile neutropenic inpatients reported similar efficacy of oral ciprofloxacin plus amoxicillin/clavulanate vs. an IV regimen (ceftazidime or ceftriaxone plus amikacin) [55, 56]. Ciprofloxacin monotherapy provides suboptimal coverage for gram-positive organisms including viridans group streptococci [57]. Levofloxacin is more active against gram-positive bacteria but less active than ciprofloxacin against *Pseudomonas* [58, 59]. A randomized trial ($N = 333$) reported similar efficacy (80 % vs. 82 %) of oral moxifloxacin compared to oral ciprofloxacin plus amoxicillin/clavulanate. Neurologic events were more common with moxifloxacin, and diarrhea was more common with the combination therapy [60].

Antibacterial therapy in low-risk patients with negative blood cultures is continued for at least two afebrile days after ANC recovery to ≥500 cells/μL or for five to seven days in the absence of myeloid reconstitution [61]. A meta-analysis of RCTs of low-risk febrile neutropenic patients reported that outpatient oral and parenteral antibiotics had similar efficacy (RR 0.93). The site of care (outpatient vs. inpatient) was not significantly associated with treatment failure (RR 0.81) [62]. The rate of hospital admission in patients receiving outpatient empiric therapy is in the range of 3–10 %.

The American Society of Clinical Oncology (ASCO) panel recommends empiric oral fluoroquinolone (ciprofloxacin or levofloxacin) plus amoxicillin/clavulanate for low-risk febrile neutropenic patients. Ciprofloxacin plus clindamycin is an alternative for penicillin-allergic patients [24, 51]. The NCCN panel recommends moxifloxacin monotherapy for patients who may not require *Pseudomonas* coverage. However, patients who have received fluoroquinolone prophylaxis before fever developed are at increased risk for infection with antibiotic-resistant strains including MRSA, vancomycin-resistant *Enterococcus* (VRE), and ESBL-producing gram-negative bacteria. These patients therefore require hospital admission and initial management with broad-spectrum parenteral antibiotics [24] (**Figure 6**).

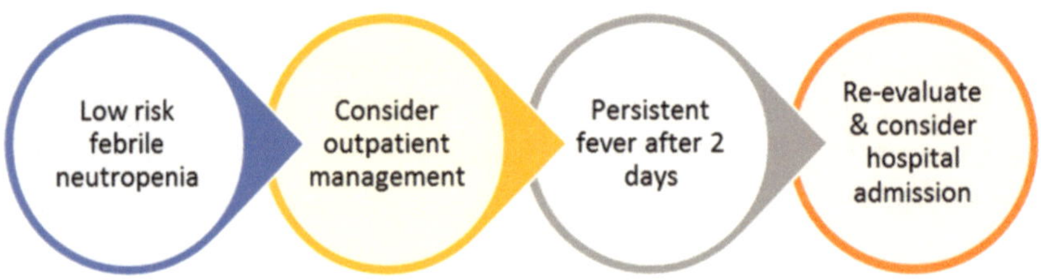

Figure 6. Management of low-risk febrile neutropenia.

4.5. Initial empiric antibacterial therapy for high-risk patients

Fever through periods of prolonged profound neutropenia during induction chemotherapy for acute leukemia or pre-engraftment phase of allogeneic HSCT may be due to serious or life-threatening infections. Febrile neutropenic patients with severe comorbidities, hepatic or renal dysfunction, or MASCC scores < 21 or in Talcott groups 1–3 are also at a high risk for infection-related complications. These patients should receive emergent evaluation, prompt resuscitation, and timely administration of broad-spectrum parenteral antibiotics to avoid progression to a sepsis syndrome and possibly death. A retrospective study of patients with severe sepsis reported decreased overall mortality (19.5 % vs. 33.2 %; $p = .02$) in patients who received antibacterial therapy within 1 h of presentation as opposed to latter [63].

The selection of initial antibacterial agent for high-risk febrile neutropenic patients is guided by clinical stability, recent antimicrobial use, medication allergy, potential site of infection, and susceptibility patterns of institutional pathogens. Empiric antibiotic regimens should have a broad spectrum (gram-positive and gram-negative coverage), bactericidal activity, antipseudomonal activity, and minimal toxicity. Current guidelines recommend initial monotherapy with antipseudomonal beta-lactam agent, such as cefepime, meropenem, imipenem-cilastatin, or piperacillin-tazobactam [16, 24]. None of these agents is superior in the empiric treatment of febrile neutropenia. However, ceftazidime monotherapy is avoided due to limited activity against viridans group streptococci and rising resistance rates among gram-negative bacteria [64].

Combination therapy is not superior to empiric monotherapy but may be associated with more adverse effects. Aminoglycoside plus antipseudomonal agent may be considered for suspected gram-negative bacteremia or sepsis syndrome or if the institution has high levels of gram-negative-resistant bacteria [65–67].

Empiric vancomycin therapy is not associated with a benefit in mortality. Nevertheless, there is concern regarding emergence of vancomycin-resistant *Enterococcus* (VRE) and *S. aureus* and increased incidence of hepatic and renal toxicity [68–71]. Current guidelines do not support its use as a routine component of the initial regimen. However, its empiric use is appropriate for suspected vascular catheter-related infection (CRI), gram-positive bacteremia, cellulitis, severe mucositis, hypotension or septic shock, pneumonia, and known colonization with MRSA or drug-resistant *Streptococcus pneumoniae* [72–75]. Vancomycin is usually discontinued after 48 h if cultures fail to grow resistant gram-positive organisms. In a randomized trial of febrile neutropenic patients with proven or suspected gram-positive infection (N = 611), linezolid demonstrated similar efficacy and safety when compared to vancomycin [76]. Linezolid is therefore an alternative for vancomycin-intolerant patients and vancomycin-resistant gram-positive pathogens. Myelosuppression may limit its use in patients with compromised bone marrow function.

Neutropenic sepsis is a major cause of mortality. Diagnostic criteria include altered mental status, systolic hypotension of ≤100 mm Hg, and tachypnea of >22 breaths/min. These patients should receive aggressive resuscitation and monitoring in an intensive care unit. Patients in septic shock require vasopressors to maintain mean arterial pressure (MAP) ≥ 65 mm Hg despite adequate fluid resuscitation and have a lactate level >2 mmol/L. Stress-dose steroids (50 mg hydrocortisone every six hours for 5–7 days) may benefit those with ongoing hypotension (systolic blood pressure <90 mm Hg for more than 1 h) refractory to fluid resuscitation and vasopressor support [77]. RCTs of patients with severe sepsis demonstrated that high-dose steroids (>300 mg hydrocortisone per day) increased overall mortality and the risk of secondary infections [78–81]. The initial empiric antimicrobial regimen should include a broad-spectrum beta-lactam plus aminoglycoside plus vancomycin. In addition, antifungal agents such as fluconazole or an echinocandin may be strongly considered.

The empiric broad-spectrum antibacterial should be continued until the patient is afebrile for at least 2 days and the ANC is ≥500 cells/μL on at least one occasion but is showing a consistent increasing trend. Documented infections should be managed with appropriate antimicrobials based on blood culture and susceptibility results. High-risk patients with persistent unexplained fever despite 3–5 days of antibacterial therapy should undergo assessment for undiagnosed fungal infection. Empiric coverage for *Candida* and/or for molds should also be considered (**Figure 7**).

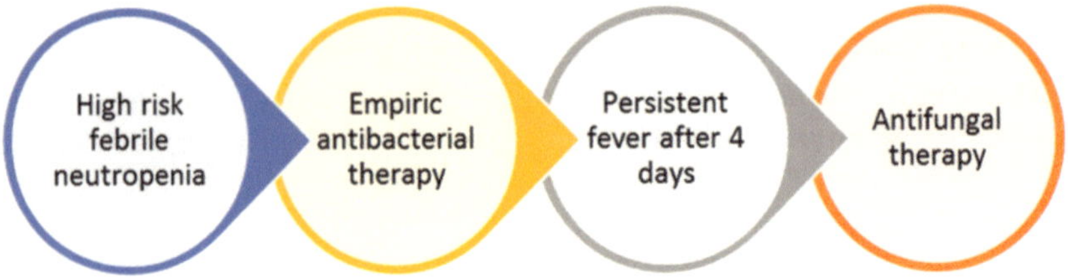

Figure 7. Management of high-risk febrile neutropenia.

4.6. Empiric antifungal therapy

Persistent fever refers to an episode of fever during neutropenia that does not resolve after 4 days of broad-spectrum antibacterial agents. *Recurrent fever* refers to a new episode of fever during neutropenia that occurs >2 days after resolution of a first fever while continuing broad-spectrum antibacterial therapy. Patients with prolonged neutropenia with persistent or recurrent fever are at increased risk for life-threatening infections with yeasts or molds. Early detection of these invasive fungal diseases (IFDs) is challenging because of limited sensitivity and specificity of clinical presentation and investigative modalities. As an example, the mere isolation of *Candida* spp. from sputum, urine, or stool samples ascertains colonization only and is not indicative of invasive infection requiring treatment [82].

Definitive diagnosis of IFD requires histological evidence of deep tissue invasion or positive culture from normally sterile sites. Whereas histopathology has the ability to make organism-specific diagnoses in only a few cases, the results of fungal cultures may not be available in a timely fashion for clinical decisions. Furthermore, repeated biopsies and microbiologic samplings may be difficult to obtain in critically ill neutropenic patients. Although molecular diagnostics have the potential for increased sensitivity and a rapid turnaround time, it lacks the ability to differentiate invasive infection from colonization or contamination. The detection of fungal-specific antibodies also does not consistently differentiate between previous exposure and active disease.

Fungal antigen detection assays target components of the fungal cell wall that are shed during fungal growth. The β-(1-3)-ᴅ glucan (BDG) test detects *Candida*, *Aspergillus*, *Pneumocystis*, and *Fusarium* species in serum specimens. It has a sensitivity of 63–90 % and specificity greater than 95 %. False-positive results may occur in patients on hemodialysis and those receiving intravenous immunoglobulin. The galactomannan (GM) assay detects *Aspergillus* species in both serum and bronchoalveolar lavage (BAL) specimens. It has a sensitivity of 70–89 % and specificity of 85–92 % in patients with hematologic malignancies [83]. BAL testing is more sensitive than serum testing in patients with invasive pulmonary aspergillosis [84]. False-positive results have been noted with other filamentous fungi. While the BDG assay is capable of detecting a broad range of fungi, both serum BDG and GM assays have similar sensitivities for *Aspergillus* species [85].

"Empiric" antifungal coverage is administered to patients without an identified fever source.

Two RCTs of patients with persistent febrile neutropenia showed that the addition of empiric amphotericin B (on day 4 of fever or on day 7) to continued antibacterial regimen reduced the frequency of IFD [86, 87]. Initiation of antifungal agents after 4–7 days of persistent fever thus became the standard of care. Amphotericin B (AMB) use is limited by infusion reactions and renal toxicity. Subsequent studies have therefore focused on identifying safer and equally effective alternatives. Lipid formulations of amphotericin B (L-AMB) are as effective but less nephrotoxic [88]. Fluconazole lacks activity against molds (*Aspergillus* spp.) [89, 90]. Itraconazole has similar efficacy as AMB but less toxicity [91]. It should be used with caution in patients with reduced ejection fraction or heart failure. Intravenous formulation is not available in the United States. Erratic oral bioavailability precludes its use as an empiric agent. Voriconazole is superior to L-AMB (fewer breakthrough fungal infections). Isavuconazole is non-inferior to voriconazole with improved tolerability and safety. Caspofungin has similar efficacy as L-AMB (**Figure 8**).

Author	N	Study drugs		Response Rate %		IFI%	
		Arm 1	Arm 2	Arm 1	Arm 2	Arm 1	Arm 2
Walsh TJ [102]	687	AMB	L-AMB	49	50	8.7	5.0
Boogaerts M [103]	384	AMB	Itraconazole	38	47	2.7	2.7
Walsh TJ [104]	937	L-AMB	Voriconazole	31	26	5.0	1.9 $p<0.05$
Walsh TJ [105]	1095	L-AMB	Caspofungin	34	34	4.3	5.2

Figure 8. Alternatives to empirical amphotericin B (AMB); L-AMB, lipid formulations of amphotericin B.

"Preemptive" antifungal treatment is administered only when the evidence of IFD is suggested by positive fungal biomarker and/or high-resolution imaging (CT chest/sinus) results. In a meta-analysis of nine published studies of high-risk patients presenting with persistent febrile neutropenia, diagnostic-driven strategy significantly reduced antifungal use (RR 0.48, 95 % CI 0.27–0.85) and cost without increasing IFD-related mortality (RR 0.82, 95 % CI 0.36–1.87) or overall mortality (RR 0.95, 95 % CI 0.46–1.99) [92]. *Candida* and *Aspergillus* are the most common fungal pathogens causing invasive disease. The widespread use of azole prophylaxis has substantially decreased the incidence of invasive candidiasis (IC) in comparison to *Aspergillus* and other molds. Serum BDG test is a useful screening tool for both *Candida* and *Aspergillus* species. The Fungitell (BDG) assay has a positive cutoff value of >80 pg/mL. Though a negative test result does not rule out the diagnosis of IFD, a false-positive result may occur in patients with mucositis whose gastrointestinal tract is colonized with *Candida*. Serum GM (cutoff optical density index [ODI] > 0.5) is the current gold standard for detection of invasive aspergillosis (IA). The sensitivity of this assay is significantly reduced in patients receiving anti-mold prophylaxis. Combining BG and GM assays improves the diagnosis of IA [93].

Aspergillus DNAemia may precede the release of fungal GM into the bloodstream. However, *Aspergillus* polymerase chain reaction (PCR) testing has not been widely implemented due to a lack of standardization. A randomized trial reported that combined serum GM and *Asper-*

gillus PCR monitoring leads to an earlier diagnosis of invasive aspergillosis [94]. A meta-analysis of thirteen studies ($N = 1670$) showed that the absence of serum GM and *Aspergillus* PCR-positive test may obviate the need for antifungal agents with a negative predictive value of 100 % [95].

The echinocandins (caspofungin, micafungin, and anidulafungin) are fungicidal against most *Candida* spp. with similar efficacy [96–99]. Voriconazole is the treatment of choice for invasive aspergillosis. Isavuconazole is non-inferior to voriconazole with fewer side effects [100].

The European Organization for Research and Treatment of Cancer (EORTC) is completing accrual ($N = 556$) of a phase 3 prospective trial (NCT01288378) comparing empiric and preemptive caspofungin therapy in patients with AML or MDS. The results of this study should clarify the utility of diagnostic testing and the efficacy of preemptive strategies in patients receiving antifungal prophylaxis with fluconazole (**Figures 9** and **10**).

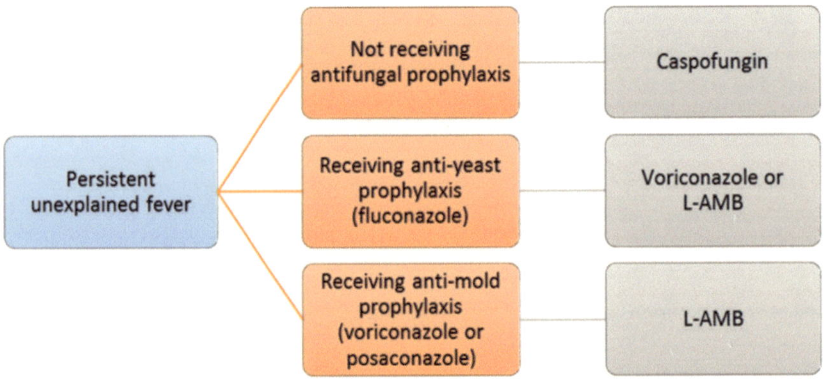

Figure 9. Management of persistent febrile neutropenia. L-AMB, lipid formulations of amphotericin B.

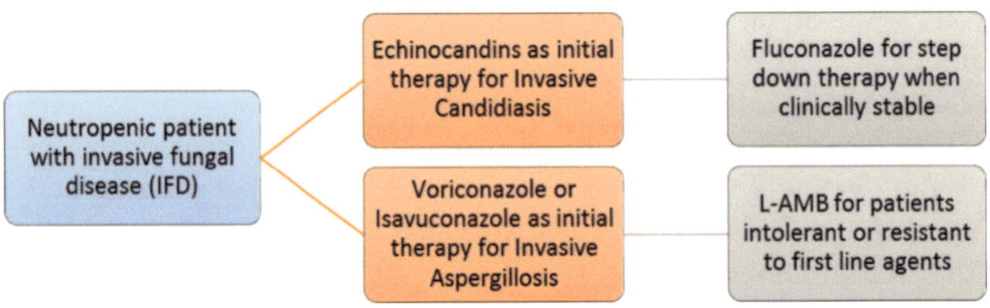

Figure 10. Management of febrile neutropenia with invasive fungal disease. L-AMB, lipid formulations of amphotericin B.

4.7. Vascular catheter–related infections

Central venous catheters (Hickman or Mediport) are frequently used in patients undergoing cancer treatment. Neutropenic patients are at increased risk for vascular catheter–related

http://dx.doi.org/10.5772/64372

infections (CRI). The hub/lumen of the catheter is the major site of colonization and source of infection. The differential time to positivity (DTP) of 120 min or more between centrally and peripherally drawn blood cultures is indicative of catheter-related bacteremia. Common pathogens include coagulase-negative *staphylococci, S. aureus,* and *Candida* spp.

Febrile neutropenic patients with clinical signs of CRI should receive empiric antipseudomonal beta-lactam agent plus vancomycin. Catheter removal should be strongly considered for tunnel or port-pocket infections; septic phlebitis; septic shock; endocarditis; bacteremia due to *S. aureus, P. aeruginosa,* or *Candida* spp.; and persistent bloodstream infection despite ≥72 h of therapy. Catheter removal is not required for coagulase-negative *staphylococci* bacteremia. Antimicrobial therapy is modified after availability of blood culture and susceptibility results. Antibacterial agents should be administered for a minimum of 14 days following catheter removal and clearance of blood cultures. Prolonged treatment for 4–6 weeks is recommended for bacteremia complicated with deep tissue infection, endocarditis, septic thrombosis, or persistent bacteremia or fungemia occurring >72 h after catheter removal [24].

5. Refining infection control during cancer care

Preventing infection in cancer patients is a comprehensive initiative led by Centers for Disease Control and Prevention to reduce infections in patients with cancer. PreventCancerInfections.org is a website that provides information about neutropenia, signs and symptoms of infections, and methods to control them. Basic infection control and prevention plan is a tool for outpatient oncology facilities that outlines infection control policies and procedures. Standard precautions refer to the minimum measures to prevent infection including hand and respiratory hygiene, proper use of gowns and gloves, injection safety, medication storage and handling, and cleaning and disinfection of devices and environmental surfaces. Transmission-based precautions supplement standard precautions when managing potentially infectious patients. Medical providers should perform hand hygiene before and after contact with the patients. The examination room should be cleaned and disinfected before using it for another patient.

Home infection prevention measures include avoiding contact with sick people or sharing personal items, keeping household surfaces clean, consuming clean and properly cooked food, and practicing good oral, dental, and skin hygiene. Patients should be instructed to contact their provider immediately in the event of fever, redness, swelling, or drainage from surgical and vascular catheter sites. Annual influenza vaccination with the inactivated virus is recommended for all caregivers.

High-risk patients with febrile neutropenia require hospital admission. Allogeneic HSCT recipients should be confined in private rooms with >12 air exchanges/h and high-efficiency particulate air filtration. Non-transplant patients do not require a private room. Household pets, fresh flowers, and plants should not be allowed in the rooms [24]. Patients should take daily showers, maintain good health hygiene, and eat well-cooked foods. Rectal thermometers, enemas, suppositories, and rectal examinations should be avoided during periods of neutropenia. Healthcare workers and visitors with symptomatic infections should avoid contact with the neutropenic patient. Hospitals should conduct periodic risk assessment of multidrug-resistant organism acquisition and transmission.

6. Conclusions

Infection is an important cause of morbidity and mortality in cancer patients. Febrile neutropenia is a frequent and expensive complication of myelosuppressive chemotherapy. Evidence-based guidelines provide strong recommendations for the empiric management of initial fever and persistent fever. The management of febrile patients receiving anti-yeast or anti-mold prophylaxis is still evolving. The best management of recurrent fever remains unanswered. Judicious use of antimicrobial prophylaxis is an important infection prevention strategy. Hand hygiene, contact precautions, and disinfecting patient-care equipment remain crucial approaches for preventing the spread of infections in medical facilities. The repertoire of new medications for the treatment of cancer is continually expanding. Physicians should be vigilant of the immunosuppressive potential and the risk of opportunistic infections associated with the use of these newer biologics.

Author details

Deepjot Singh[1,3*] and Robert A. Bonomo[2,3]

*Address all correspondence to: deepjot.singh@case.edu

1 Hematology Oncology, Medical Service, Louis Stokes Cleveland Department of Veterans Affairs Medical Center, Cleveland, USA

2 Infectious Diseases Sections, Medical Service, Louis Stokes Cleveland Department of Veterans Affairs Medical Center, Cleveland, USA

3 Department of Medicine, Case Western Reserve University, Cleveland, USA

References

[1] Preventing Infections in Cancer Patients. Centers for Disease Control. Nov. 19, 2015. Retrieved from http://www.cdc.gov/cancer/dcpc/resources/features/PreventInfections/index.htm

[2] Dinan MA, Hirsch BR, Lyman GH. Management of chemotherapy-induced neutropenia: measuring quality, cost, and value. J Natl Compr Canc Netw. 2015;13(1):e1–e7.

[3] Saral R, Burns WH, Prentice HG. Herpes virus infections: clinical manifestations and therapeutic strategies in immunocompromised patients. Clin Haematol. 1984;13:645–660.

[4] Funakoshi T, Suzuki M, Muss HB. Infection risk in breast cancer patients treated with trastuzumab: a systematic review and meta-analysis. Breast Cancer Res Treat. 2015;149(2):321–330.

[5] Garcia CA, Wu S. Risk of serious infection with mTOR inhibitors everolimus and temsirolimus in the treatment of cancer: a meta-analysis of randomized controlled trials. J Clin Oncol. 2014;32s:35s.

[6] Ma Q, Gu LY, Ren YY, et al. Increased risk of severe infections in cancer patients treated with vascular endothelial growth factor receptor tyrosine kinase inhibitors: a meta-analysis. Onco Targets Ther. 2015;8:2361–2374.

[7] Sandherr, M, Hentrich, M, von Lilienfeld-Toal, M. Antiviral prophylaxis in patients with solid tumours and haematological malignancies—update of the Guidelines of the Infectious Diseases Working Party (AGIHO) of the German Society for Hematology and Medical Oncology (DGHO). Ann Hematol. 2015;94(9): 1441–1450.

[8] Mitka M. FDA: increased HBV reactivation risk with ofatumumab or rituximab. JAMA. 2013;310(16):1664.

[9] Huang H, Li X, Zhu J, et al. Entecavir vs lamivudine for prevention of hepatitis B virus reactivation among patients with untreated diffuse large B-cell lymphoma receiving R-CHOP chemotherapy: a randomized clinical trial. JAMA. 2014;312:2521–2530.

[10] Bradley AM, Devine M, DeRemer D. Brentuximab vedotin: an anti-CD30 antibody-drug conjugate. Am J Health Syst Pharm. 2013;70(7):589–597.

[11] Darzalex (Daratumumab). Package insert, https://www.janssenmd.com/pdf/darzalex/DARZALEX_PI.pdf

[12] Montillo M, Ricci F, Miqueleiz S, et al. Alemtuzumab in the treatment of fludarabine refractory B-cell chronic lymphocytic leukemia (CLL). Biologics. 2008;2(1):41–52.

[13] Markham A. Elotuzumab: first global approval. Drugs. 2016;76(3):397–403.

[14] Harrison C, Mesa R, Ross D, et al. Practical management of patients with myelofibrosis receiving ruxolitinib. Expert Rev Hematol. 2013;6(5):511–523.

[15] Santos FP, Verstovsek S. Efficacy of ruxolitinib for myelofibrosis. Expert Opin Pharmacother. 2014;15(10):1465–1473.

[16] National Comprehensive Cancer Network (NCCN). Clinical Practice Guidelines in Oncology. Prevention and treatment of cancer-related infections. Version 2. 2015. http://www.nccn.org (Accessed on February 12, 2016).

[17] Engels EA, Lau J, Barza M. Efficacy of quinolone prophylaxis in neutropenic cancer patients: a meta-analysis. J Clin Oncol. 1998;16:1179–1187.

[18] Gafter-Gvili A, Fraser A, Paul M, et al. Antibiotic prophylaxis for bacterial infections in afebrile neutropenic patients following chemotherapy. Cochrane Database Syst Rev. 2012;1:CD004386.

[19] Bucanev G, Micozzi A, Menichetti F, et al. Levofloxacin to prevent bacterial infection in patients with cancer and neutropenia. N Engl J Med. 2005;353:977–987.

[20] Cullen M, Steven N, Billingham L, et al. Antibacterial prophylaxis after chemotherapy for solid tumors and lymphomas. N Engl J Med. 2005;353 (10):988.

[21] Razonable R, Litzow MR, Khaliq Y, et al. Bacteremia due to viridans group Streptococci with diminished susceptibility to Levofloxacin among neutropenic patients receiving levofloxacin prophylaxis. Clin Infect Dis. 2002;34(11):1469–1474.

[22] Cook PP, Catrou P, Gooch M, et al. Effect of reduction in ciprofloxacin use on prevalence of methicillin-resistant *Staphylococcus aureus* rates within individual units of a tertiary care hospital. J Hosp Infect. 2006;64(4):348–351.

[23] Loo VG, Poirier L, Miller MA, et al. A predominantly clonal multi-institutional outbreak of *Clostridium difficile*-associated diarrhea with high morbidity and mortality. N Engl J Med. 2005;353:2442–2449.

[24] Freifeld AG, Bow EJ, Sepkowitz KA, et al. Clinical practice guideline for the use of antimicrobial agents in neutropenic patients with cancer: 2010 Update by the Infectious Diseases Society of America. Infectious Diseases Society of America, Clin Infect Dis. 2011;52(4):e56.

[25] Rotstein C, Bow EJ, Laverdiere M, et al. Randomized placebo-controlled trial of fluconazole prophylaxis for neutropenic cancer patients: benefit based on purpose and intensity of cytotoxic therapy. The Canadian Fluconazole Prophylaxis Study Group. Clin Infect Dis. 1999;28:331–340.

[26] Koh LP, Kurup A, Goh YT, et al. Randomized trial of fluconazole versus low-dose amphotericin B in prophylaxis against fungal infections in patients undergoing hematopoietic stem cell transplantation. Am J Hematol. 2002;71:260–267.

[27] Ethier MC, Science M, Beyene J, et al. Mould-active compared with fluconazole prophylaxis to prevent invasive fungal diseases in cancer patients receiving chemotherapy or haematopoietic stem-cell transplantation: a systematic review and metaanalysis of randomised controlled trials. Br J Cancer. 2012;106(10):1626–1637.

[28] Vardakas KZ, Michalopoulos A, Falagas ME. Fluconazole versus itraconazole for antifungal prophylaxis in neutropenic patients with haematological malignancies: a meta-analysis of randomised-controlled trials. Br J Haematol. 2005;131(1): 22–28.

[29] Wang J, Zhan P, Zhou R, et al. Prophylaxis with itraconazole is more effective than prophylaxis with fluconazole in neutropenic patients with hematological malignancies. Med Oncol. 2010;27(4):1082–1088.

[30] Marks DI, Pagliuca A, Kibbler CC, et al. IMPROVIT Study Group. Voriconazole versus itraconazole for antifungal prophylaxis following allogeneic haematopoietic stem-cell transplantation. Br J Haematol. 2011;155(3):318–327.

[31] Cornely OA, Maertens J, Winston DJ, et al. Posaconazole vs. fluconazole or itraconazole prophylaxis in patients with neutropenia. N Engl J Med. 2007;356(4):348–359.

[32] Mattiuzzi GN, Alvarado G, Giles FJ, et al. Open-label, randomized comparison of itraconazole versus caspofungin for prophylaxis in patients with hematologic malignancies. Antimicrob Agents Chemother. 2006;50(1):143–147.

[33] Wingard JR, Carter SL, Walsh TJ, et al. Blood and Marrow Transplant Clinical Trials Network. Randomized, double-blind trial of fluconazole versus voriconazole for prevention of invasive fungal infection after allogeneic hematopoietic cell transplantation. Blood. 2010;116(24):5111–5118.

[34] Huang X, Chen H, Han M, et al. Multicenter, randomized, open-label study comparing the efficacy and safety of micafungin versus itraconazole for prophylaxis of invasive fungal infections in patients undergoing hematopoietic stem cell transplant. Biol Blood Marrow Transplant. 2012;18(10):1509–1516.

[35] Ullmann AJ, Lipton JH, Vesole DH, et al. Posaconazole or fluconazole for prophylaxis in severe graft-versus-host disease. N Engl J Med. 2007;356(4):335–347.

[36] Chaftari AM, Hachem RY, Ramos E, et al. Comparison of posaconazole versus weekly amphotericin B lipid complex for the prevention of invasive fungal infections in hematopoietic stem-cell transplantation. Transplantation. 2012;94(3):302–308.

[37] Stern A, Green H, Paul M, et al. Prophylaxis for Pneumocystis pneumonia (PCP) in non-HIV immunocompromised patients. Cochrane Database Syst Rev. 2014;10:CD005590.

[38] Marras TK, Sanders K, Lipton JH, et al. Aerosolized pentamidine prophylaxis for *Pneumocystis carinii pneumonia* after allogeneic marrow transplantation. Transpl Infect Dis. 2002;4(2):66–74.

[39] Sangiolo D, Storer B, Nash R, et al. Toxicity and efficacy of daily dapsone as *Pneumocystis jiroveci* prophylaxis after hematopoietic stem cell transplantation: a case-control study. Biol Blood Marrow Transplant. 2005;11(7):521–529.

[40] Eliakim-Raz N, Vinograd I, Zalmanovici TA, et al. Influenza vaccines in immunosuppressed adults with cancer. Cochrane Database Syst Rev. 2013;10:CD008983.

[41] Lorry R, Myron L, Per L, et al. 2013 IDSA clinical practice guideline for vaccination of the immunocompromised host. Clin Infect Dis. 2014;58(3):e44–e100.

[42] Engelhard D, Mohty B, de la Camara R, et al. European guidelines for prevention and management of influenza in hematopoietic stem cell transplantation and leukemia patients: summary of ECIL-4 (2011), on behalf of ECIL, a joint venture of EBMT, EORTC, ICHS, and ELN. Transpl Infect Dis. 2013;15:219–232.

[43] Reddy KR, Beavers KL, Hammond SP, et al. American Gastroenterological Association I. American Gastroenterological Association Institute guideline on the prevention and treatment of hepatitis B virus reactivation during immunosuppressive drug therapy. Gastroenterology. 2015;148:215–219, quiz e16–e17.

[44] Marinone C, Mestriner M. HBV disease: HBsAg carrier and occult B infection reactivation in haematological setting. Dig Liver Dis. 2011;43(Suppl 1):S49–S56.

[45] Zaia J, Baden L, Boeckh MJ, et al. Viral disease prevention after hematopoietic cell transplantation. Bone Marrow Transplant. 2009;44(8):471–482.

[46] Yahav D, Gafter-Gvili A, Muchtar E, et al. Antiviral prophylaxis in haematological patients: systematic review and meta-analysis. Eur J Cancer. 2009;45(18):3131–3148.

[47] Keating M, Coutré S, Rai K, et al. Management guidelines for use of alemtuzumab in B-cell chronic lymphocytic leukemia. Clin Lymphoma. 2004;4(4):220–227.

[48] Erard V, Guthrie KA, Varley C et al. One-year acyclovir prophylaxis for preventing varicella-zoster virus disease after hematopoietic cell transplantation: no evidence of rebound varicella-zoster virus disease after drug discontinuation. Blood. 2007;110(8): 3071–3077.

[49] Tomblyn M, Chiller T, Einsele H, et al. Guidelines for preventing infectious complications among hematopoietic cell transplantation recipients: a global perspective. Biol Blood Marrow Transplant. 2009;15(10):1143.

[50] George B, Pati N, Gilroy N, et al. Pre-transplant cytomegalovirus (CMV) serostatus remains the most important determinant of CMV reactivation after allogeneic hematopoietic stem cell transplantation in the era of surveillance and preemptive therapy. Transpl Infect Dis. 2010;12(4):322–329.

[51] Flowers CR, Seidenfeld J, Bow EJ et al. Antimicrobial prophylaxis and outpatient management of fever and neutropenia in adults treated for malignancy: American Society of Clinical Oncology Clinical Practice Guideline. JCO. 2013;31(3):794–810.

[52] Talcott JA, Siegel RD, Finberg R et al. Risk assessment in cancer patients with fever and neutropenia: a prospective, two-center validation of a prediction rule. J Clin Oncol. 1992;10:316–322.

[53] Klastersky J, Paesmans M, Rubenstein EB et al. The Multinational Association for Supportive Care in Cancer risk index: a multinational scoring system for identifying low-risk febrile neutropenic cancer patients. J Clin Oncol. 2000;18(16): 3038–3051.

[54] Kamana M, Escalante C, Mullen CA, et al. Bacterial infections in low-risk, febrile neutropenic patients. Cancer. 2005;104(2):422–426.

[55] Freifeld A, Marchigiani D, Walsh T, et al. A double-blind comparison of empirical oral and intravenous antibiotic therapy for low-risk febrile patients with neutropenia during cancer chemotherapy. N Engl J Med. 1999;341(5):305–311.

[56] Kern WV, Cometta A, De Bock R, et al. Oral versus intravenous empirical antimicrobial therapy for fever in patients with granulocytopenia who are receiving cancer chemotherapy. International Antimicrobial Therapy Cooperative Group of the European Organization for Research and Treatment of Cancer. N Engl J Med. 1999;341(5):312–318.

[57] Kerr KG, Armitage HT, McWhinney PH. Activity of quinolones against viridans group streptococci isolated from blood cultures of patients with haematological malignancy. Support Care Cancer. 1999;7(1):28–30.

[58] Gasink LB, Fishman NO, Weiner MG, et al. Fluoroquinolone-resistant *Pseudomonas aeruginosa*: assessment of risk factors and clinical impact. Am J Med. 2006;119:526.e19–526.e25.

[59] Kaye KS, Kanafani ZA, Dodds AE, et al. Differential effects of levofloxacin and ciprofloxacin on the risk for isolation of quinolone-resistant *Pseudomonas aeruginosa*. Antimicrob Agents Chemother. 2006;50:2192–2196.

[60] Kern WV, Marchetti O, Drgona L, et al. Oral antibiotics for fever in low-risk neutropenic patients with cancer: a double-blind, randomized, multicenter trial comparing single daily moxifloxacin with twice daily ciprofloxacin plus amoxicillin/clavulanic acid combination therapy—EORTC infectious diseases group trial XV. J Clin Oncol. 2013;31(9):1149–1156.

[61] de Naurois J, Novitzky-Basso I, Gill MJ, et al. Management of febrile neutropenia: ESMO Clinical Practice Guidelines. Ann Oncol. 2010;21 (Suppl 5):v252–v256.

[62] Teuffel O, Ethier MC, Alibhai SM, et al. Outpatient management of cancer patients with febrile neutropenia: a systematic review and meta-analysis. Ann Oncol. 2011;22(11): 2358–2365.

[63] Gaieski DF, Mikkelsen ME, Band RA, et al. Impact of time to antibiotics on survival in patients with severe sepsis or septic shock in whom early goal-directed therapy was initiated in the emergency department. Crit Care Med. 2010;38:1045–1053.

[64] Tunkel AR, Sepkowitz KA. Infections caused by viridans streptococci in patients with neutropenia. Clin Infect Dis. 2002;34(11):1524–1529.

[65] Cometta A, Zinner S, de Bock R, et al. Piperacillin-tazobactam plus amikacin versus ceftazidime plus amikacin as empiric therapy for fever in granulocytopenic patients with cancer. The International Antimicrobial Therapy Cooperative Group of the

European Organization for Research and Treatment of Cancer. Antimicrob Agents Chemother. 1995;39(2):445–452.

[66] Cordonnier C, Herbrecht R, Pico JL, et al. Cefepime/amikacin versus ceftazidime/amikacin as empirical therapy for febrile episodes in neutropenic patients: a comparative study. The French Cefepime Study Group. Clin Infect Dis. 1997;24(1):41–51

[67] Flaherty JP, Waitley D, Edlin B et al. Multicenter, randomized trial of ciprofloxacin plus azlocillin versus ceftazidime plus amikacin for empiric treatment of febrile neutropenic patients. Am J Med. 1989;87(5A):278S–282S.

[68] Edmond MB, Ober JF, Weinbaum DL, et al. Vancomycin-resistant *Enterococcus faecium* bacteremia: risk factors for infection. Clin Infect Dis. 1995;20(5):1126–1133.

[69] Montecalvo MA, Shay DK, Patel P, et al. Bloodstream infections with vancomycin-resistant enterococci. Arch Intern Med. 1996;156(13):1458–1462.

[70] Vancomycin added to empirical combination antibiotic therapy for fever in granulocytopenic cancer patients. European Organization for Research and Treatment of Cancer (EORTC) International Antimicrobial Therapy Cooperative Group and the National Cancer Institute of Canada-Clinical Trials Group. J Infect Dis. 1991;163(5):951–958.

[71] Lin MY, Hayden MK. Methicillin-resistant *Staphylococcus aureus* and vancomycin-resistant enterococcus: recognition and prevention in intensive care units. Crit Care Med. 2010;38(8 Suppl):S335–S344.

[72] Mermel LA, Allon M, Bouza E, et al. Clinical practice guidelines for the diagnosis and management of intravascular catheter-related infection: 2009 Update by the Infectious Diseases Society of America. Clin Infect Dis. 2009;49(1):1–45

[73] Dellinger RP, Levy MM, Carlet JM, et al. Surviving Sepsis Campaign: international guidelines for management of severe sepsis and septic shock: 2008. Intensive Care Med. 2008;34(1):17–60.

[74] Kaul DR, Collins CD, Hyzy RC. New developments in antimicrobial use in sepsis. Curr Pharm Des. 2008;14(19):1912–1920.

[75] Daum RS. Clinical practice. Skin and soft-tissue infections caused by methicillin-resistant *Staphylococcus aureus*. N Engl J Med. 2007;357(4):380–390.

[76] Jaksic B, Martinelli G, Perez-Oteyza J, et al. Efficacy and safety of linezolid compared with vancomycin in a randomized, double-blind study of febrile neutropenic patients with cancer. Clin Infect Dis. 2006;42(5):597–607.

[77] Patel GP, Balk RA. Systemic steroids in severe sepsis and septic shock. Am J Respir Crit Care Med. 2012;185:133–139.

[78] Veterans Administration Systemic Sepsis Cooperative Study Group. Effect of high-dose glucocorticoid therapy on mortality in patients with clinical signs of systemic sepsis. N Engl J Med. 1987;317(11):659–665.

[79] Bone RC, Fisher CJ Jr, Clemmer TP, et al. A controlled clinical trial of high-dose methylprednisolone in the treatment of severe sepsis and septic shock. N Engl J Med. 1987;317(11):653–658.

[80] Cronin L, Cook DJ, Carlet J, et al. Corticosteroid treatment for sepsis: a critical appraisal and meta-analysis of the literature. Crit Care Med. 1995;23(8):1430–1439.

[81] Slotman GJ, Fisher CJ Jr, Bone RC, et al. Detrimental effects of high-dose methylprednisolone sodium succinate on serum concentrations of hepatic and renal function indicators in severe sepsis and septic shock. The Methylprednisolone Severe Sepsis Study Group. Crit Care Med. 1993;21(2):191–195.

[82] Cornely OA, Bassetti M, Calandra T, et al. ESCMID* guideline for the diagnosis and management of Candida diseases 2012: non-neutropenic adult patients. Clin Microbiol Infect. 2012;18(Suppl 7):19–37.

[83] Pfeiffer CD, Fine JP, Safdar N. Diagnosis of invasive aspergillosis using a galactomannan assay: a meta-analysis. Clin Infect Dis. 2006;42(10):1417–1427

[84] Fisher CE, Stevens AM, Leisenring W, et al. Independent contribution of bronchoalveolar lavage and serum galactomannan in the diagnosis of invasive pulmonary aspergillosis. Transpl Infect Dis. 2014;16(3):505–510.

[85] Marty FM, Koo S. Role of (1–3)-beta-d-glucan in the diagnosis of invasive aspergillosis. Med Mycol. 2009;47(Suppl 1):S233–S240.

[86] Pizzo PA, Robichaud KJ, Gill FA, et al. Empiric antibiotic and antifungal therapy for cancer patients with prolonged fever and granulocytopenia. Am J Med. 1982;72(1):101–111.

[87] Empiric antifungal therapy in febrile granulocytopenic patients. EORTC International Antimicrobial Therapy Cooperative Group. Am J Med. 1989;86(6Pt1):668–672.

[88] Walsh TJ, Finberg RW, Arndt C, et al. Liposomal amphotericin B for empirical therapy in patients with persistent fever and neutropenia. National Institute of Allergy and Infectious Diseases Mycoses Study Group. N Engl J Med. 1999;340(10):764–771.

[89] Viscoli C, Castagnola E, Van Lint MT, et al. Fluconazole versus amphotericin B as empirical antifungal therapy of unexplained fever in granulocytopenic cancer patients: a pragmatic, multicentre, prospective and randomised clinical trial. Eur J Cancer. 1996;32A(5):814–820.

[90] Winston DJ, Hathorn JW, Schuster MG, et al. A multicenter, randomized trial of fluconazole versus amphotericin B for empiric antifungal therapy of febrile neutropenic patients with cancer. Am J Med. 2000;108(4):282–289.

[91] Boogaerts M, Winston DJ, Bow EJ, et al. Intravenous and oral itraconazole versus intravenous amphotericin B deoxycholate as empirical antifungal therapy for persistent fever in neutropenic patients with cancer who are receiving broad-spectrum antibacterial therapy. A randomized, controlled trial. Ann Intern Med. 2001;135(6):412–422.

[92] Fung M, Kim J, Marty FM, et al. Meta-analysis and cost comparison of empirical versus pre-emptive antifungal strategies in hematologic malignancy patients with high-risk febrile neutropenia. PLoS ONE. 2015;10(11):e0140930. doi: 10.1371/journal.pone.0140930

[93] Pazos, C, Ponton J, Del Palacio A. Contribution of (1→3)-β-d-glucan chromogenic assay to diagnosis and therapeutic monitoring of invasive aspergillosis in neutropenic adult patients: a comparison with serial screening for circulating galactomannan. J Clin Microbiol 2005;43:299–305.

[94] Aguado JM, Vasquez L, Fernandez-Ruiz M, et al. Serum galactomannan versus a combination of galactomannan and polymerase chain reaction-based Aspergillus DNA detection for early therapy of invasive aspergillosis in high-risk hematological patients: a randomized controlled trial. Clin Infect Dis. 2015;60:405–414. doi: 10.1093/cid/ciu833. pmid: 25336623

[95] Arvanitis M, Anagnostou T, Mylonakis E. Galactomannan and polymerase chain reaction-based screening for invasive aspergillosis among high-risk hematology patients: a diagnostic meta-analysis. Clin Infect Dis. 2015;61(8):1263–1272.

[96] Mora-Duarte J, Betts R, Rotstein C, et al. Comparison of caspofungin and amphotericin B for invasive candidiasis. N Engl J Med. 2002;347(25):2020–2029.

[97] Kuse ER, Chetchotisakd P, da Cunha CA, et al. Micafungin versus liposomal amphotericin B for candidaemia and invasive candidosis: a phase III randomized double-blind trial. Lancet. 2007;369(9572):1519–1527.

[98] Reboli AC, Shorr AF, Rotstein C, et al. Anidulafungin compared with fluconazole for treatment of candidemia and other forms of invasive candidiasis caused by *Candida albicans*: a multivariate analysis of factors associated with improved outcome. BMC Infect Dis. 2011;11:261–269.

[99] Pappas PG, Rotstein CM, Betts RF, et al. Micafungin versus caspofungin for treatment of candidemia and other forms of invasive candidiasis. Clin Infect Dis. 2007;45(7):883–893.

[100] Maertens J, Patterson TF, Rahav G, et al. A phase 3 randomized, double-blind trial evaluating isavuconazole vs voriconazole for the primary treatment of invasive fungal disease caused by Aspergillus spp. or other filamentous fungi (SECURE). 24th ECCMID. Barcelona, Spain, 10–13 May, 2014.

http://dx.doi.org/10.5772/64372

[101] Walsh TJ, Pappas P, Winston DJ, et al. Voriconazole compared with liposomal amphotericin B for empirical antifungal therapy in patients with neutropenia and persistent fever. N Engl J Med. 2002;346(4):225–234.

[102] Walsh TJ, Teppler H, Donowitz GR, et al. Caspofungin versus liposomal amphotericin B for empirical antifungal therapy in patients with persistent fever and neutropenia. N Engl J Med. 2004;351(14):1391–1402.

Chapter 5

Nutrition and Indirect Calorimetry

Danish Ahmad, Kellie Joseph and
Christopher Halpin

Additional information is available at the end of the chapter

http://dx.doi.org/10.5772/64385

Abstract

Nutrition support is important in the care of patients with both acute and chronic illness. Optimizing nutritional support for the critically ill and patients with acute and chronic respiratory disorders has been shown to shorten length of stay, shorten duration of mechanical ventilation, lower health-care costs and reduce morbidity and mortality while improving functional quality of life. Nutritional requirements are difficult to predict in patients diagnosed with cancer due to their disease processes, altered inflammatory responses and metabolic rates among many other variables. Often predictive equations are used to estimate energy requirements and the average dietary energy intake needed to maintain energy balance. Energy requirements can be estimated through the use of over 200 predictive equations. Utilization of indirect calorimetry as the 'gold standard' for measuring resting metabolic rate (RMR) and resting energy expenditure (REE) can provide support in all states of health and disease. This chapter will identify and discuss the role of indirect calorimetry, examine the reasons why indirect calorimetry is more reliable than predictive equations in determining a patient's calorie requirement, and when it is most applicable to incorporate indirect calorimetry measurements in the care of cancer patients.

Keywords: indirect calorimetry, nutrition, resting energy expenditure, predictive equations, critical illness

1. Introduction

Nutritional support is important in the care of patients with acute and chronic illness. Up to 50% of hospitalized patients are clinically malnourished, which is associated with increased infectious morbidity, increased hospital length of stay and mortality [1]. Optimizing nutritional support of the critically ill and patients with acute and chronic respiratory disorders reduces morbidity and mortality, shortens hospital length of stay, shortens duration of mechanical ventilation, and lowers health-care costs while improving functional quality of life. Energy needs vary according to activity level and state of health and can vary greatly particularly in the critically ill, malnourished, postoperative and infected population. Nutritional requirements are difficult to predict in cancer patients in particular because of altered inflammatory responses and metabolic rates caused by the disease process itself. Siobal and Baltz describe a functional nutrition support system to include an interdisciplinary team approach for assessment and treatment, which incorporates an evaluation of nutritional risk, standards for nutritional support, an appropriate assessment and reassessment process, proper implementation, route of support based on patient condition, and a means of measuring nutrient requirements to determine whether target goals are being met [2].

Inflammation associated with disease/injury can cause anorexia and alterations in body composition and stress metabolism. Predominantly cytokine mediated; persists as long as the inflammatory stimulus is present. These metabolic alterations include elevated energy expenditure, lean tissue catabolism (proteolysis), fluid shift to the extracellular compartment, acute phase protein changes, and decreased synthesis of serum albumin, transferrin and prealbumin. This leads to clinical deterioration of lean body mass, poor wound healing, increased risk of nosocomial infection, weakened respiratory muscles, impaired immunity, organ dysfunction, and increased morbidity and mortality. Several studies have shown that metabolically stressed and malnourished patients have more negative outcomes and higher health-care costs. Patients with continuous energy deficits have a higher ventilator-dependence rate, longer intensive care unit (ICU) stay, and higher mortality [3–6].

2. Calorimetry

Calorimetry is a process that quantifies the heat release from metabolism of cellular fuels. It provides assessment of caloric energy present in foods and allows for measurement of energy expenditure to determine adequate calorie requirement. This information can be used for a myriad of clinical applications. Evaluating appropriate caloric intake, avoidance of overfeeding and underfeeding, and measuring caloric requirements in different disease states can be achieved through calorimetry.

It can be measured in a direct as well as an indirect manner. Direct calorimetry measures actual heat release from the metabolism of foods. This was carried out *ex vivo*. Indirect calorimetry measures metabolism of foods *in vivo*. Direct calorimetry is a challenging process that requires technical proficiency. Turell and Alexander [7] demonstrated that indirect calorimetry measurements of energy expenditure are accurate within 0.6–0.7% to direct calorimetry. In this section, the advent, mechanisms, technicalities, and limitations of indirect calorimetry are discussed.

Indirect calorimetry is able to provide information regarding metabolic rate, energy expenditure, and anaerobic thresholds. This technique has been around since late nineteenth century

http://dx.doi.org/10.5772/64385

[8]. Since then various advancements have been made in this field. With these advancements, it is becoming a staple of clinical medicine, particularly in the assessment of adequate caloric intake.

Indirect calorimetry measures respiratory gas exchange and estimates energy production [9]. Initially, mathematical equations modeled the metabolism of carbohydrates and lipids. These stoichiometric equations include oxygen as a reactant in conjunction with carbohydrates, or lipids. The products of this reaction are carbon dioxide and water, with heat as a byproduct.

$$1\text{g Lipid} + 2.029\text{L}O_2 \leftrightarrow 1.43\text{L}CO_2 + 1.09\text{g}H_2O \ [9] \quad (1)$$

$$1\text{g Glucose} + 0.746\text{L } O_2 \leftrightarrow 0.746\text{L}CO_2 + 0.6\text{g}H_2O \ [9] \quad (2)$$

The heat produced from these reactions can be written as

$$\text{Heat output} = 3.9(VO_2) + 1.1(VCO2) \times 1.44 \ [10] \quad (3)$$

VO_2 = oxygen consumption in ml/min

VCO_2 = carbon dioxide production in ml/min

1440 min/day, 1000 cal/kcal

Extracting chemical energy from cellular fuels is accomplished by completely oxidizing the substrate to carbon dioxide and water [9]. The ratio of CO_2 production to oxygen consumption is referred to as the respiratory quotient (RQ) [9]. RQ is VCO_2/VO_2 at the cellular level which is difficult to measure. Respiratory exchange ratio (RER) is VCO_2/VO_2 measured from expired air. Under steady-state conditions, the blood and gas transport systems are keeping pace with tissue metabolism, thus RER can be used as index of metabolic events and assumed to be equivalent to RQ. The test was carried out when subjects are resting. During rest, the system is noted to be under steady state. Assumptions believed to be true during indirect calorimetry measurement, aside from RER = RQ, are that growth is not occurring, interconversion of fuels are not occurring, and anaerobic metabolism is not occurring as it is only accurate for steady-state oxidative metabolism.

3. Protein metabolism

Measurement of protein metabolism was thought to be to clinically challenging through indirect calorimetry. In early 1900s, assumptions were made that a fixed percentage of total calories arise from the metabolism of protein, and the contribution could be ignored without effecting the estimations of energy expenditure [10]. This assumption was based on analysis of various regional diets worldwide and that on average humans consume 10–15% of their total calories as proteins [10, 11].

However, ignoring the contribution of protein metabolism does add a degree of error to the calculations. Per Turell and Alexander, a systemic error of 1.0% is introduced for each 12.3% increment in protein contribution to the total oxidative state. Varying the degree of protein intake does change the basal metabolic rate [12].

In 1948, Weir demonstrated calculations that allowed for protein metabolism to be included.

The nitrogen backbone present in all proteins is metabolized through various pathways in the human body. About 80% of nitrogen is eliminated through the kidneys as urea [13]. Hence, measuring urea excretion allows for calculation of dietary protein intake. Weir demonstrated that quantifying urinary nitrogen over a 24-hour period could then be modeled in an equation to measure contribution of protein metabolism. Hence, the equation can be written as below:

$$1\text{g Protein} + 0.966\text{L } O_2 \leftrightarrow 0.782\text{L}CO_2 + 0.45\text{g}H_2O \text{ [9]} \tag{4}$$

As nitrogen is noted to be 16% of protein by weight, the subsequent equation can be written:

$$1\,\text{g Protein} = 6.25\,\text{Urine Nitrogen} \tag{5}$$

The heat produced from combination of these fuel substrates can be written as:

$$\text{Heat output} = 3.9(VO_2) + 1.1(VCO_2) - 2.17(\text{Urine Nitrogen}) \times 1.44 \text{ [10]} \tag{6}$$

With these comprehensive changes, the RQ for various metabolic fuels can be provided.

RQ	Carbohydrate	Protein	Fat
	1	0.802 [14]	0.718 [15]

Normal RQ values range between 0.67 and 1.2 while results outside of this range are suggestive of technical errors.

4. Calorimeters

Specific device and corresponding instruments are used for indirect calorimetry. The several technologies that are available require precise calibration and measurements of volume and gas analysis. The traditional device used for decades was the Deltatrac and subsequently the Deltatrac II [16]. It is the set gold standard for indirect calorimetry. Since then, other products have become available. The Quark resting metabolic rate (RMR) and CCMexpress are two such devices.

The Quark RMR metabolic meter is developed by COSMED. It is a European company based out of Italy. Quark RMR measures VO_2, VCO_2, and resting energy expenditure (REE). It is also able to distinguish the different substrates being utilized. It can measure these values on spontaneously and mechanically ventilated patients.

The CCM express metabolic meter is developed by MGC diagnostics, an American company. This device also measures REE in the usual manner. It is able to perform these measurements even when inspired oxygen concentrations are above 60%, as well as with fluctuating oxygen concentrations.

These new products have been compared to the Deltatrac II, as the acknowledged gold standard. Validation trials have been performed to certify the reproducibility of these calorimeters [17–19]. Other trials have not shown similar results. The variance between the Deltatrac II and these other calorimeters has been higher than clinically acceptable [16]. The disagreement between these new calorimeters requires for further refinements for them to be used in clinical practice. These machines need to demonstrate fidelity to the set gold standard in multiple clinical settings. These settings include spontaneously breathing as well as mechanically ventilated patients. The mechanically ventilated patients are the critically sick ones [16, 20].

The M-COVX is a metabolic meter that can be fully integrated into a mechanical ventilation circuit. It is manufactured by the Deltatrac parent company [21].

MedGem is a metabolic meter that measures VO_2 alone. It makes an assumption on RQ and is for use in spontaneously ventilated patients [21].

5. Methodology

These calorimeters can be used in spontaneously breathing or mechanically ventilated patients. The inspired gas can be room air or a supplemental oxygen mixture. In a spontaneously breathing patient, an overlying canopy, face tent, or facemask can be used for gas collection. A mouthpiece with a nose clip can also be used. In mechanically ventilated patients, the calorimeter can be attached to the ventilator system. The total expired gas volume is recorded for calculations [21–25].

The several technologies that are available require precise calibration and measurements of volume and gas analysis. Although indirect calorimeters are easy to operate and understand, there are several variables that can impact accuracy in measurements. All of the devices contain gas analyzers and a flow/volume measuring device. Gas analyzers must be responsive and capable of measuring minimal changes in oxygen enriched and room air environments. The ability to measure minute changes in gas concentrations as small as 0.001% while the flow/volume measurements must be accurate across the expected clinical range is a requirement of these devices.

The principle of Haldane transformation assumes that nitrogen (N_2) is an insoluble gas and does not participate gas exchange. As a consequence, it is constant in both inspired and expired volumes. Assuming that oxygen (O_2) and carbon dioxide (CO_2) are the only gases exchanged in the lungs the inspired volume can be calculated from the expired volume [21].

Calorimeters measure inspired O_2 and CO_2 concentration, expired O_2 and CO_2 concentration, and expired gas volume. With the use of Haldane transformation, REE can be provided through indirect calorimetry. As previously stated, measuring at steady-state approximates REE to RQ.

Steady state is described as a patient under resting conditions. Many factors can effect achievement of these conditions (**Table 1**). They include but are not limited to patients undergoing physical stress such as fever and pain. Patients should be resting in a quiet room without excess environmental stimuli. Changes in the environment around the patient also affect these results [26].

30-min rest period prior (III)	Measure while room temp b/t 72–77°F (II)
Not engage in any activity during said period (V)	Measure in a quiet room (V)
For the duration of RER measurement, disregard first 5 min and then continue for at least 4 min with <10% coefficient of variation in VO_2 and $VCO_2$and <5% for RQ (III)	At least 4 h without stimulants and 140 min without smoking (III)
Measure while supine (II)	Measure after a 7-h fast (III)
Any device ok for gas collection (III)	At least 12–48 h after light-to-vigorous exercise (V)
Measure any time of day (III)	At least 30 min rest after light activity (III)
	If RQ < 0.67 or >1.3, assume error and repeat (II)

The Academy of Nutrition and Dietetics utilizes a grading system for determining strength of evidence of studies and reports based on five factors. These factors are quality, consistency, quantity, clinical impact, and generalizability. The grading system is as follows: (I) Good, (II) Fair, (III) Limited, (IV) Expert Opinion only, and (V) Grade not assigned [27].

Table 1. Best practices for performing indirect calorimetry in healthy and non critically ill patients.

There are three areas that can pose challenges during the technical performance of indirect calorimetry. These are patient interface, elevated oxygen concentrations, and variability of mechanical ventilators. One interface for spontaneously breathing at rest subjects is a large canopy that encompasses the patients head and shoulders (**Figure 1**). This must be adapted to the subject and be free of potential leaks to prevent the loss of exhaled air. The canopy is designed to ensure collection of exhaled air close to the subjects mouth yet spacious enough for comfort and visibility. There is also an interface of a large form fitting mask that has open slots for adequate flow circulation. Another type of mask fitting is shown here (**Figure 2**). Each manufacturer identifies the ideal interface that will work well with their systems.

Many authors have described in detail about the effects of elevated oxygen on the VO_2 measurement. Branson describes an 1% error in FiO_2 measurement at 0.40 results in a 15% error in VO_2 measurement. An error effect comes into play when the FiO_2 is close to 1, and the denominator of the Haldane equation (1-FiO_2) approaches zero [28]. The impact of these variables on data results is noted in **Table 2** [28].

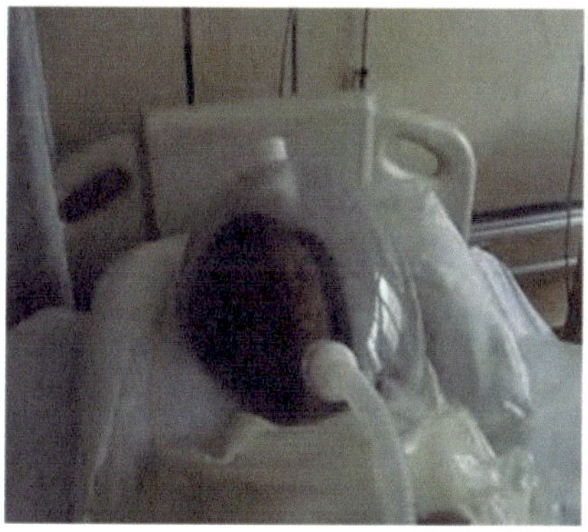

Figure 1. Carefusion canopy.

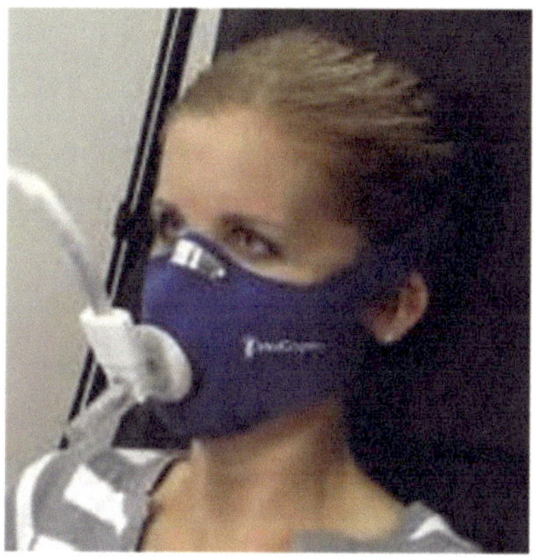

Figure 2. MedGraphics interface.

	VO_2	VCO_2	REE	RQ
Leaks	Low	Low	Low	Unchanged
Unstable FiO_2	Low or high	Unchanged	Low or high	Low or high
FiO_2 > 80%*	Low or high	Unchanged	Low or high	Low or high
Mixing of inspired and expired gas (active exhalation valve)	Normal or high	Low	Normal or low	Low

*VO_2 measurements are highly suspected.

Table 2. Effect of ventilator operation and ventilation issues on REE and RQ.

Performances of indirect calorimetry on subjects who are mechanically ventilated have less potential for system leaks. This closed system provides a simplified way to collect exhaled gas, and the measurement of inspired gas can be determined easily at the inspiratory limb of a ventilator circuit. The problems that arise in indirect calorimetry during mechanical ventilation are fluctuations in FiO_2, ventilator mode, and flow requirements. The variability in FiO_2 occurs due to increased flow demands, bias flow to provide better patient interface, and high minute ventilation. Leaks can occur during mechanical ventilation due to unsealed airways or incompetent tracheal cuffs, through chest tubes or bronchopleural fistulas. Other technical aspects to consider during mechanical ventilation also include: calibration errors, recent changes in ventilator settings that may not reflect steady state, moisture in the system, patient-ventilator dyssynchrony, and acute hyperventilation or hypoventilation (impact physiologic CO_2).

Equipment variables and methodology of measuring gas concentrations can lead to inaccurate results as well. At the point of data accumulation, the issue becomes how to decrease the variance in collected data points. The variance can be due to differences in tidal volume, respiratory rate, and other patient factors [8]. These variations can lead to changes in VO_2 and VCO_2 measurements.

In order to eliminate these data variations, several techniques have been developed. They include breath averaging, time averaging, and digital filtering [8].

Breath averages collect data points over a predefined number of breaths. The average of these data points is used as the final result. Similarly, time averaging is the collection of data points over pre-designated period of time. The data accrued from all of the breaths during the pre-designated period are averaged to give one value [8].

Digital filtering removes data points that are not within a range of the median data points. In this instance, setting the range in any one direction can drastically alter the results. If the range is too high, then data points that are not necessarily precise can be included in the calculations and yield a higher/lower value than accepted. If the range is noted to be too low then many data points that are valid can be excluded from the analysis and thus providing distorted data values [8].

Recommendations exist to add correction factor estimates to decrease the error in indirect calorimetry as well. Patients can be defined as hypometabolic, hypermetabolic, and normal. Correction factors can be added for dietary thermogenesis. This is the energy required for metabolism of food. Other common correction factors are activity factors and spontaneous ventilation [29]. Recent trials are not in complete agreement with this practice. Some clinicians advocate for the removal of correction factors. They contend that correction factors lead to overfeeding. Over feeding has known deleterious outcomes in patients and this should be avoided [29]. This issue is important when dealing with patient in respiratory distress. Over feeding will lead to an increase in RQ and subsequently an increase in minute ventilation. Patients in respiratory distress will need to increase their minute ventilation at a time of respiratory compromise. This scenario is often seen in patients on mechanical ventilation. These patients will be excess nutrition that leads to them having an increase in their baseline minute ventilation. When the time comes for spontaneous breathing trials to assess their readiness for spontaneous ventilation, they fail these trials as a consequence of overfeeding.

6. Interpretation

Measurement of indirect calorimetry is best performed with the patient at rest with a goal of achieving steady state. Steady state is characterized by <5% change from baseline measurements of the respiratory quotient (RQ), and 10%, respectively, for the VO_2 (oxygen uptake) and Ve (minute ventilation) during data collection. Nutrition, whether parental or enteral feeding, need not be held. It is recommended that the subject be at rest with minimal distractions or disturbances. Most studies consider 20–30 min of data collection an accurate reflection of 24-hour energy expenditure. Some literature also supports an abbreviated time of 5 min of steady-state data.

7. Predictive equations

While indirect calorimetry remains the gold standard for caloric assessment, predictive equations provide an alternate method of determining nutritional requirements. Given the expense associated with indirect calorimetry and advanced training required to perform accurate metabolic studies, as well as limited availability of equipment, predictive equations are a cost-effective strategy for broadly assessing metabolic requirements.

The Harrison-Benedict equation (HBE) is the most established method dating back to 1919, from studies conducted in healthy, young volunteers to assess resting energy expenditure (REE). Thus, application of these formulas in the critical care setting, particularly in the elderly, should be with caution. While utilization of these equations remains widespread, it has been noted that they may a results in a significant error in estimating REE. There have been subsequent studies attempting to refine the degree of error since the development of these equations [30, 31].

The Mifflin-St. Jeor (MSJ) equation was developed through multiple regression analyses utilizing indirect calorimetry data in a cohort of healthy men and women, encompassing a wider array of age and weights not taken into consideration in the original HBE [30, 31]. The Ireton-Jones is another equation that has been validated in trials. It has been more recently developed. It included mechanical ventilation, trauma, burns, and obesity as factors during its development and hence is more likely to be valid in these specific clinical settings [32].

Tatucu-Babet *et al.* looked at 2349 publications with 18 studies included. One hundred and sixty variations of 13 predictive equations were reviewed. Thirty-eight percent underestimated and 12% overestimated energy expenditure by more than 10% at the group level. On an individual level, the equations underestimated and overestimated energy expenditure in 13–90% and 0–88% of patients, respectively. Differences of up to 43% below and 66% above indirect calorimetry values were observed at the patient level [33].

A criticism of predictive equations is the accuracy of application to the heterogeneous critically ill patient population. These patients have continual metabolic change, which increases the difficulty of finding one prediction equation that will be accurate across the spectrum. Accuracy of these equations varies significantly, ranging from approximately 40 to 70%, where accuracy is defined as within 10% of the measured resting energy expenditure [34]. However, without the common availability of indirect calorimetry, they remain a valuable tool for widespread baseline understanding of nutritional requirement. The equation selected should be used with patients similar to the reference population from which the equation was derived.

8. Indirect calorimetry and respiratory failure

In critically ill patients, in particular those with respiratory failure, the assessment of adequate nutrition is paramount. Respiratory muscle strength begins to decline after a few days of suboptimal nutrition [35]. Supplemental nutrition and overfeeding can increase oxygen consumption and carbon dioxide production, which can have deleterious consequences in patients with a limited ability to augment their ventilation. This can result in the need for mechanical ventilation and may make ventilatory management and weaning difficult. In a study of 213 ventilator-dependents patients, approximately 25% received calories within 10% of measured energy expenditure; 32–93% were overfed, and 12–36% were underfed [36]. Patients' energy needs predicted from equations compared to those measured via IC were 2× as likely to develop a negative energy balance associated with longer ventilator dependence [37]. An increasing RQ significantly correlated with increased respiratory rate and decreasing tidal volume, indicating rapid-shallow breathing and ventilatory compromise [38]. Adequate feeding significantly correlates with duration of ventilator dependence ($r = 0.494$, $p = 0.03$) and ICU stay ($r = 0.525$, $p = 0.02$) [39].

9. Indirect calorimetry and malignancy

There are limited studies of indirect calorimetry in the cancer population, especially with respects to the critically ill patient population. Garcia-Peris *et al.* looked prospectively at changes in resting energy expenditures measured by indirect calorimetry in patients with head and neck cancers treated with chemoradiation. They found the REE changed significantly. Compared to the Harris-Benedict equation, REE was represented by a U-shaped curve over time, as compared to a decreasing line by Harris-Benedict. Further, Harris-Benedict significantly underestimated REE before and at the end of treatment [40]. Reeves *et al.* looked at resting energy expenditures in solid tumor patients undergoing therapy. They found the fat-free, mass-adjusted REE was not significantly different between cancer patients and healthy patients, and the limits of agreement were wide for all prediction methods, up to 40% below and 30% above measured REE [41]. Johnson *et al.* compared measured and predicted resting energy expenditures in 33 cancer patients divided in weight-stable and weight-losing groupings. They found no difference in measured REE between the groups. However, the Harris-Benedict equation predicted REE was within clinical acceptable limits for only 61% of weight-losing and 56% of weight-stable patients, respectively [42].

In those patients with malignancy and critical illness, the accuracy of the predictive equations may be even more skewed, as this specific patient population has not been well studied. Further, the metabolic demands of a patient may be affected by cancers of different sites-of-origin, different cancer cell subtypes, different stages of disease, as well as a history of prior/ongoing chemotherapy and radiotherapy. As such, indirect calorimetry at an individual point and trended over time may be a more accurate reflection of one's nutritional needs.

Author details

Danish Ahmad[2], Kellie Joseph[1*] and Christopher Halpin[1]

*Address all correspondence to: kellie.joseph@ctca-hope.com

1 Cancer Treatment Center of America – ERMC, Philadelphia, USA

2 Hahnemann University Hospital, Philadelphia, USA

References

[1] ASPEN Board of Directors and the Clinical Guidelines Task Force. Guidelines for use of parental and enteral nutrition in adult and pediatric patients. JPEN J Parenter Enteral Nutr. 2002;26(1 Suppl):1SA–138SA.

[2] Siobal, M,Baltz, J. A guide to the nutritional assessment and treatment of the critically ill patient. AARC. 2013; 1–45.

[3] Bassili H, Deitel M. Effects of nutritional support on weaning patients off mechanical ventilators. J Parenteral Nutr. 1981;5(2):161–163.

[4] Villet S, Chiolero RL, Bollmann MD, Revelly J, Cayeux M, Delarue J, et al. Negative impact of hypocaloric feeding and energy balance on clinical outcome in ICU patients. Clin Nutr. 2005;24(4):502–509.

[5] Askanazi J, Starker PM, Olsson C, Hensle TW, Lockhart SH, Kinney JM, et al. Effect of immediate postoperative nutritional support on length of hospitalization. Ann Surg. 1986;203(3):236–239.

[6] Bartlett RH, Dechert RE, Mault JR, Ferguson SK, Kaiser AM, Erlandson EE. Measurement of metabolism in multiple organ failure. Surgery. 1982;92(4):771–779.

[7] Turell DJ, Alexander JK. Experimental evaluation of Weir's formula for estimating metabolic rate in man. JAppl Physiol. 1964; 19: 946–8.

[8] Robergs RA, Dwyer D, Astorino T. Recommendations for improved data processing from expired gas analysis indirect calorimetry. Sports Med. 2010; 40 (2): 95–111. doi: 10.2165/11319670-000000000-00000.

[9] Ferrannini E. The theoretical bases of indirect calorimetry: a review. Metabolism. 1988; 37 (3):287–301.

[10] Weir JB. New methods for calculating metabolic rate with special reference to protein metabolism. J Physiol. 1949; 109 (1–2): 1–9.

[11] McCance RA, Widdowson EM. The digestability of English and Canadian wheats with special reference to the digestability of wheat protein by man. J Hyg (Lond). 1947; 45 (1): 59–64.

[12] Wishart GM. The influence of the protein intake on the basal metabolism. J Physiol. 1928; 65 (3): 243–54.

[13] Even PC, Nadkarni NA. Indirect calorimetry in laboratory mice and rats: principles, practical considerations, interpretation and perspectives. Am J Physiol Regul Integr Comp Physiol. 2012; 303 (5): R459–76. doi:10.1152/ajpregu.00137.2012.

[14] Lusk G. The elements of the science of nutrition. 4th ed. W. B. Saunders Co., Philadelphia and London: 1928.

[15] Cathcart EP, Cuthbertson DP. The composition and distribution of the fatty substances of the human subject. J Physiol.1931; 72 (3): 349–60.

[16] Graf S, Karsegard VL, Viatte V et al. Comparison of three indirect calorimetry devices and three methods of gas collection: a prospective observational study. ClinNutr.2013; 32 (6): 1067–72. doi:10.1016/j.clnu.2013.08.012.

[17] Ashcraft CM, Frankenfield DC. Validity test of a new open-circuit indirect calorimeter. J Parenter Enteral Nutr. 2015; 39 (6): 738–42. doi:10.1177/0148607114526242.

[18] Sundstrom M, Tjader I, Rooyackers O et al. Indirect calorimetry in mechanically ventilated patients. A systematic comparison of three instruments. ClinNutr.2013; 32 (1): 118–21. doi:.1016/j.clnu.2012.06.004.

[19] Blond E, Maitrepierre C, Normand S et al. A new indirect calorimeter is accurate and reliable for measuring basal energy expenditure, thermic effect of food and substrate oxidation in obese and healthy subjects. E Spen Eur E J Clin Nutr Metab. 2011; 6 (1): e7–e15.

[20] Graf S, Karsegard VL, Viatte V et al. Evaluation of three indirect calorimetry devices in mechanically ventilated patients: which device compares best with the Deltatrac II? A prospective observational study. Clin Nutr.2015; 34 (1): 60–5. doi:10.1016/j.clnu. 2014.01.008.

[21] da Roche EE, Alves VG, da Fronseca RB. Indirect calorimetry: methodology, instruments and clinical application. Curr Opin Clin Nutr Metab Care. 2006; 9 (3): 247–56.

[22] Haugen HA, Melanson EL, Tran ZV et al. Variablity of measured resting metabolic rate. Am J Clin Nutr. 2003; 78 (6): 1141–5.

[23] Grunwald GK, Melanson EL, Forster JE et al. Comparison of methods for achieving 24-hour energy balance in a whole-room indirect calorimeter. Obes Res. 2003; 11 (6): 752–9.

[24] Forse RA. Comparison of gas exchange measurements with a mouthpiece, face mask, and ventilated canopy. JPEN J Parenter Enteral Nutr. 1993; 17 (4): 388–91.

[25] Isbell TR, Klesges RC, Meyers AW et al. Measurement reliability and reactivity using repeated measurements of resting energy expenditure with a face mask, mouthpiece, and ventilated canopy. JPEN J Parenter Enteral Nutr. 1991; 15 (2): 165–8.

[26] Wooley JA, Sax HC. Indirect calorimetry: applications to practice. Nutr Clin Pract. 2003; 18 (5): 434–9.

[27] Fullmer S et al. Evidence analysis library review of best practices for performing indirect calorimetry in healthy and non–critically ill individuals. J Acad Nutr Diet. 2015; 115 (9):1417–46.

[28] Branson, R, Rodrigeuz, J, Tajchman, S, Wooley, J. Critical decisions: enhancing patient-specific care in the critically ill. 2012; Saxe Healthcare Communications: 1–12.

[29] Holdy KE. Monitoring energy metabolism with indirect calorimetry: instruments, interpretation, and clinical application. Nutr Clin Pract. 2004; 19 (5): 447–54.

[30] Segadilha NL, Rocha EE, Tanaka LM et al. Energy expenditure in critically ill elderly patients: indirect calorimentry vs predictive equations. JPEN J Parenter Enteral Nutr. 2016; Jan 29 pii:0148607115625609.

[31] Picolo MF, Lago AF, Menegueti MG et al. Harris-Benedict equation and resting energy expenditure estimates in critically ill ventilator patients. Am J Crit Care. 2016; 25 (1): E21–9. doi:10.4037/ajcc2016758.

[32] Ireton-Jones CS, Turner WW Jr, Liepa GU et al. Equations for the estimation of energy expenditures in patients with burns with special reference to ventilator status. J Burn Care Rehabil. 1992; 13 (3): 330–3.

[33] Tatucu-Babet OA et al. The prevalence of underprescription or overprescription of energy needs in critically ill mechanically ventilated adults as determined by indirect calorimetry: asystematic literature review. JPEN J Parenter Enteral Nutr. 2016;40(2): 212–25.

[34] Walker RN, Heuberger RA. Predictive equations for energy needs for the critically ill. Respir Care. 2009; 54(4): 509–21.

[35] Fraser IM. Effects of refeeding on respiration and skeletal muscle function. Clin Chest Med. 1986;7(1):131–139.

[36] McClave SA, Lowen CC, Kleber MJ, Nicholson JF, Jimmerson SC, McConnell JW, et al. Are patients fed appropriately according to their caloric requirements? JPEN J Parenteral Enteral Nutr. 1998;22(6):375–381.

[37] McClave SA, Snider HL, Ireton-Jones C. Can we justify continued interest in indirect calorimetry? (editorial) Nutr Clin Pract. 2002;17(3):133–136.

[38] McClave SA et al. Clinical use of the respiratory quotient from indirect calorimetry. JPEN J Parenteral Enteral Nutr. 2003; 27(1): 21–26.

[39] Kan MN, Chang HH, Sheu WF, Cheng CH, Lee BJ, Huang YC. Estimation of energy requirements for mechanically ventilated, critically ill patients using nutritional status. Crit Care. 2003;7(5):R108–R115.

[40] Garcia-Peris et al. Prospective study of REE changes in head and neck cancer pts treated with chemoradiotherapy measured by indirect calorimetry. Nutrition. 2005; 21:1107–1112.

[41] Reeves M. et al. Resting energy expenditure in patient with solid tumors undergoing anticancer therapy. Nutrition. 2006; 22:609–615.

[42] Johnson G. et al. Cancer cachexia: measured and predicted resting energy expenditures for nutritional needs evaluation. Nutrition. 2008; 24:443–450.

Chapter 6

Management of Pain, Agitation, and Delirium in Mechanically Ventilated Oncology Patients

Trisha Patel and Mark E. Lewis

Additional information is available at the end of the chapter

http://dx.doi.org/10.5772/64268

Abstract

Attention has heightened over the last several years to the importance of managing pain, agitation, and delirium in mechanically ventilated patients due to the multiple long-term adverse effects patients experience after an intensive care unit (ICU) admission. Furthermore, clinical practice is being molded not just by the guidelines and randomized controlled trials, but also by the information gathered from real patient experiences to improve care at the bedside. The literature continues to remain sparse for providing guidance specifically in the oncology population. Therefore, several resources have been combined to better assist clinicians on making sound decisions for keeping patients comfortable on the ventilator while recognizing the differences in treatment that may need to be employed due to these patients' medical condition.

Keywords: Ventilation, Pain, Agitation, Delirium, Sedation

1. Introduction

One of the leading causes of an intensive care unit (ICU) admission is acute respiratory failure where approximately 44–69% of patients with malignancies requiring mechanical ventilation due to the progression of cancer or chemotherapy toxicity [1]. Improved survival of critically ill oncology patients has been due to the advances in the treatment of malignancies and more appropriate triage of patients for ICU admission [2]. Thus, not all families of intubated patients are met with discussions for end of life or hospice care of their loved one. Goals of weaning and extubation to allow the resumption of cancer treatment have become more common.

There is a potential increase in number of oncology patients that clinicians will manage on mechanical ventilation in the future. Therefore, the need for appropriate protocols to treat pain, agitation, and delirium is especially crucial for a population on chronic pain and anxiety medications prior to admission. However, national guidelines published by the Society of Critical Care Medicine (SCCM) in 2013 were primarily based on data from the nononcology population, which poses challenges in applying such concepts to these patients. Such protocol outcomes lack support from clinical trials in oncology patients. Studies involving ICU patients with cancer have largely focused on mortality outcomes, rather than improvement of care, due to these patients' overall poor prognosis. Thus, the concepts described in the SCCM guidelines must be applied simultaneously with literature on effective treatment of pain and agitation in noncritically ill oncology patients.

In addition to clinical trials, patient interviews conducted in the ICU are gaining more attention to help the clinician better predict the needs of the patient on mechanical ventilation. A prospective study, conducted in a medical ICU, evaluated the symptom experience of patients with a present or past diagnosis of cancer admitted during an 8-month period. The patients expressed the procedures associated with the greatest pain or discomfort were endotracheal suctioning, endotracheal and nasogastric tubes, mechanical ventilation, arterial puncture, and turning. The aspects of the environment reported to be most stressful were inability to communicate, communicate, sleep disturbances, and limited family visitation hours [2]. In this study, patients still experienced significant discomfort despite liberal administration of opioids and sedatives, along with the implementation of palliative care recommendations. This could be explained by the challenge of accurately assessing pain in mechanically ventilated patients, as well as the rate in which patients felt their stress was not relived by medications. For these reasons, it is imperative that a multidisciplinary team acquires a consistent and universal method by which these patients' pain, agitation, and delirium are managed. More importantly, the clinicians should have a strong understanding of the pharmacology of opioids and sedatives to ensure the safest agents are chosen.

2. Pain

The prevalence of pain has not been shown to differ between patients actively receiving anticancer treatment and those with an advanced- or terminal-phase disease. Studies have also published that on average 56–82.3% of cancer patients' pain is not adequately treated [3]. This emphasizes the importance of performing accurate and timely assessments of pain to ensure appropriate treatment. As recommended by SCCM guidelines, the gold standards for pain assessments in ICU patients are the numerical rating scale or visual analog scale (VAS) if a patient is communicative enough to express their level of pain. In some instances, such assessments can be challenging in ICU patients receiving high-dose sedatives during mechanical ventilation or those with altered level of consciousness [4]. If the patient is unable to self-report his/her pain, then the most valid and reliable assessments for pain are the behavioral pain scale (BPS) and the critical pain observation tool (CPOT) outlined in **Tables 1** and **2** [5], which are consistent with recommendations by NCCN guidelines for adult cancer pain. Vital signs alone are no longer recommended for detecting symptoms of pain. They only should be used as a cue to perform further assessments [4].

Indicator	Descriptor	Score	
Facial expression	No muscular tension observed	Relaxed, neutral	0
	Presence of frowning, brow lowering, orbit tightening, and levator contraction	Tensed	1
	All of the above facial movements plus eyelid tightly closed	Grimacing	2
Body movements	Does not move at all (does not necessarily mean absence of pain)	The absence of movements	0
	Slow, cautious movements, touching or rubbing the pain site, seeking attention through movements	Protection	1
	Pulling tube, attempting to sit up, moving limbs/ thrashing, not following commands, striking at staff, trying to climb out of bed	Restlessness	2
Muscle tension evaluation by passive flexion and extension of upper extremities	No resistance to passive movements	Relaxed	0
	Resistance to passive movements	Tense, rigid	1
	Strong resistance to passive movements, inability to complete them	Very tense or rigid	2
Compliance with the ventilator (intubated patients) OR	Alarms not activated, easy ventilation	Tolerating ventilator or movement	0
	Alarms stop spontaneously	Coughing but tolerating	1
	Asynchrony: blocking ventilation, alarms frequently activated	Fighting ventilator	2
Vocalization (extubated patients)	Talking in normal tone or no sound	Talking in normal tone or no sound	0
	Sighing, moaning	Sighing, moaning	1
	Crying out, sobbing	Crying out, sobbing	2

Table 1. Critical pain observation tool (CPOT) [5].

Chronic pain affects greater than 60% of oncology patients, with upwards of 66% experiencing failure of therapy [6]. Subsequently, the majority of these patients are opioid tolerant and on high doses of narcotics prior to being admitted. Upon ICU admission, many patients do not have oral access or have multisystem failure that can preclude them from receiving specific types of opioids. It becomes imperative that thorough medication reconciliations are performed to determine the amount of daily opioids the patient takes at home so that they can be converted to the most appropriate and safest formulation in the ICU. When performing such conversions, clinicians must consider incomplete cross tolerance if the patient is placed on an opioid they are not receiving prior to admission. Long-term exposure to one drug can result in the development of tolerance to those with similar structures. However, this tolerance is rarely complete with agents that bind to different receptors, thus the analgesic effect of the new agent is enhanced in the patient. Without appropriate conversions, the patient is at risk of withdrawal or overdose when rotating opioids. However, the heightened analgesic effect due to incomplete cross tolerance can also lead to excessive side effects such as respiratory depression, nausea, sedation, and dysphoria [7]. The total daily dose of the patient's regimen, both IV and oral, should be converted to the opioid to be initiated in the ICU using **Table 3** and reduced by 20–30% for cross intolerance. Persistent or chronic pain should be controlled using a combination of long-acting agents, either extended or sustained release oral formulations or continuous IV infusions, in conjunction with short-acting agent. Long-acting opioid typically comprises 50% of the total daily requirement [11].

Item	Description	Score
Facial expression	Relaxed	1
	Partially tightened (e.g., brow lowering)	2
	Fully tightened (e.g., eyelid closing)	3
	Grimacing	4
Upper limb movements	No movement	1
	Partially bent	2
	Fully bent with finger flexion	3
	Permanently retracted	4
Compliance with mechanical ventilation	Tolerating movement	1
	Coughing but tolerating ventilation for most of the time	2
	Fighting ventilator	3
	Unable to control ventilation	4

Table 2. Behavioral pain scale (BPS) [5].

Society of Critical Care Medicine Guidelines emphasize that many sources of pain have been identified in ICU patients related to not only surgery, trauma, burns, or cancer but also procedures. In a comparative, descriptive study, data were obtained from over 6000 patients to describe pain intensity and procedural distress. Procedures were defined as wound dressing changes, turning, tracheal suctioning, and wound drainage removal. The average pain score was 5–7, and the most distressful procedures were turning and wound care. Unfortunately, less than 20% of these patients actually received opiates before the procedures. With procedures performed so frequently in the ICU, this remains one of the areas that is poorly managed [12]. Therefore, it is highly encouraged patients are pre-treated with bolus doses of opioids.

Unrelieved pain leads to long-term negative outcomes, such as patients recalling traumatic memories of pain during their ICU admission. It has also been shown that inadequately treated pain is associated with physiological consequences such as increase in catecholamines leading to arteriolar vasoconstriction, impaired tissue perfusion, catabolic hypermetabolism resulting in hyperglycemia, lipolysis, and breakdown of muscle [4].

Drug	Oral (mg)	Parenteral (mg)
Morphine	30	10
Codeine	200	100
Oxycodone	20	n/a
Hydrocodone	30	n/a
Hydromorphone	7.5	1.5
Fentanyl	n/a	0.1
Methadone	Use ratio of 3:1 (morphine/methadone) to convert methadone to morphine equivalents and then convert to desired opioid	
Tramadol	120	100

Table 3. Opioid equianalgesic doses [8–10].

Managing pain in ICU patients, especially the mechanically ventilated, is almost always in conjunction with managing agitation and delirium. Therefore, pain can be managed more effectively and appropriately with several simple concepts employed:

1. Nurses should perform consistent and accurate pain assessments using the tools validated in ICU patients with reassessments performed after analgesics are administered to evaluate response to therapy.
2. Intermittent boluses versus continuous IV infusion strategies should be selected based on the frequency and severity of pain and/or patient's mental status. The use of patient-controlled administration (PCA) should be highly considered for patients responsive and cognitive to control delivery of boluses.
3. The type of opioid selected for each patient should be based on the drug pharmacokinetics/pharmacodynamics including any risks for altered clearance if the patient has evidence of organ dysfunction (see **Tables 4** and **5**).
4. Oral formulations should be limited to those patients with adequate gastrointestinal absorption.
5. Regional or neuraxial (spinal or epidural) modalities can be considered for postoperative analgesia.
6. Administer analgesics pre-emptively prior to procedures (i.e., chest tube removal, line insertion, turning the patient).
7. Analgesic agents should be started prior to sedative agents if there is any suspicion of pain. After sedatives are initiated, pain assessments can be harder to perform and less accurate in ensuring the patient is comfortable.
8. Pain medications should be titrated upward by 10–25% and doses selected based on the pain assessments using nursing driven scales. Opioid rotation should be considered if pain is inadequately controlled or persistent adverse effects are experienced [11].
9. Use of nursing-driven protocol with effective multidisciplinary discussions for adjustment of such medication orders should occur on a routine basis.

Analgesic	Onset (IV)	Duration of action	$t_{½}$	Dosing[1]	Common toxicities/major precautions
Fentanyl IV	1–2 min	0.1–5 h	1.5–6 h	25–100 mcg every 15 min PRN pain **Infusion:** 25–500 mcg/h	Large volume of distribution and high lipophilicity increasing risk of accumulation in tissues and sedation with prolonged infusions; less hypotension effect than morphine; accumulation with hepatic failure; rare: chest wall rigidity at high doses serotonin syndrome
Hydromorphone IV	5–15 min	4–5 h	2–3 h	0.2–0.6 mg every 15 min PRN pain **Infusion:** 0.5–5 mg/h	Alternative to fentanyl and morphine if long-acting agent is needed; accumulation in hepatic failure
Morphine IV	5–10 min	3–6 h	3–7 h	2–4 mg PRN pain **Infusion:** 2–15 mg/h	Common: bradycardia/hypotension, respiratory depression, and sedation especially at higher doses. Caution with risk of bronchospasm, histamine release, accumulation of active metabolite (3-morphine glucuronide) in renal failure that can lead to seizures
Methadone oral	1–3 days	4–6 h	8–59 h	2.5–10 mg every 8–12 h (titrated slowly every 3–5 days)	Common: prolongation of QTc, sedation Caution with multiple drug interactions; unpredictable pharmacokinetic/ pharmacodynamics; hepatic and renal failure will delay clearance. Rare: serotonin syndrome
Tramadol (for polyneuropathies as second-line agent in patients who did not respond to opioids)	1 h	9 h	6–8 h	50 mg once or twice daily titrated to max of 400 mg/day	Common: somnolence, constipation, dizziness, and hypotension. Reduce dose in renal or hepatic dysfunction; precipitates seizures in patients with history of seizures or those receiving medications that reduce seizure threshold; may increase risk of serotonin syndrome with SSRIs and SNRIs

[1]More aggressive dosing recommendations based on higher tolerance to opioids in most cancer patients. More conservative dosing is recommended for opioid-naïve patients.

PRN, as needed; $t_{½}$, half-life of elimination; SSRIs, selective serotonin reuptake inhibitors; SNRIs, serotonin and norepinephrine reuptake inhibitors; IV, intravenous; QTc, corrected QT interval.

Table 4. Comparison of most common opioids used in oncology ICU mechanically ventilated patients [4, 13–19].

2.1. Route of administration/formulation

The route of administration preferred for non-ICU patients is often oral, whereas for critically ill patients, intravenous is optimal when there is known or suspected altered gastrointestinal (GI) tract absorption. Furthermore, other routes such as intramuscular (IM), subcutaneous, or transdermal requiring systemic absorption are frequently avoided in critically ill patients due to erratic and unpredictable absorption [13]. Risks of changes in perfusion due to hemodynamic instability and fluid shifts can lead to potentiated or subtherapeutic effects.

2.2. Pharmacokinetic/pharmacodynamic properties and side effect profile

Table 4 illustrates the comparison of the most common analgesics used in ICU mechanically ventilated patients, with the exception of meperidine, which is discouraged in an ICU setting due to the high risk of neurotoxicity. Methadone is occasionally avoided due to the risk of QT prolongation, interaction with common ICU medications, and difficulty dosing. In the oncology setting, patients taking methadone at home can be encountered, and due to its multiple side effects, it should be converted to alternative opioids if the patient is unstable or lacks oral access. Methadone should not be discontinued abruptly without adequate alternative opioids initiated as replacement therapy to prevent withdrawal.

When the patient is hemodynamically unstable or has renal insufficiency, then fentanyl or hydromorphone is recommended as first line agents. Either of two agents, in addition to morphine, can be used for patients with no renal insufficiency or those who are stable [24]. Clinicians should also be cognitive of possible inadequate metabolism and/or clearance of medications in patients with renal and hepatic cancers which may not be evident by laboratory values.

2.3. Nonopioid analgesics

Opioid analgesics are most often the first line agents employed in general ICU patients with the ease of administration and ability to titrate. However, in patients with cancer, nonopioid agents provide a novel approach to better controlling their pain long term and helping to reduce opioid requirements. The WHO analgesic ladder provides guidelines for the treatment of cancer pain by suggesting a sequential three step approach based on severity of pain. Nonopioids are recommended for mild pain, weak opioids for moderate pain, and strong opioids for severe pain with fixed scheduled dosing according to the pharmacokinetic properties of the drugs. Typically, the nonopioids initiated in step 1 should be continued in conjunction with opioids added in the next step to allow for agents with different mechanisms of actions to improve analgesic control. There are several common nonopioid agents used to treat cancer pain that can be continued in an ICU if the patient has appropriate access. **Table 5** compares the various classes of nonopioid agents and pharmacokinetics as well as common toxicities of which to be aware when using such agents in the ICU setting. Other nonopioids found to effective in the oncology population are bisphosphonates for bone metastases and medicinal cannabinoids that are not encouraged in the ICU due to their unsafe profile.

Drug/Class	Onset of action	$t_{1/2}$	Dosing	Place in therapy	Common toxicities/major precautions
APAP IV	5–10 min	2.4 h	650 mg q4 h-1000 mg IV q 6 h (max 4 gm/day)	Opioid sparing effect. IV is a suitable agent for the treatment of mild to moderate pain in patients with no oral access or to assist with reaching peak levels with the first dose faster	Adjust dose with CrCl <30 mL/min or with CRRT
APAP PO	30–60 min	2 h	325–1000 mg q4–6 h (max 4 gm/day)		Risk for hepatotoxicity; use lower doses in older adults, heavy alcohol use or those who are malnourished
Ketorolac (IM/IV)	10 min	2.4–8.6 h	30 mg IM/IV, then 15–20 mg IM or IV q6 h up to 5 days (max 120 mg/day × 5 days)	Ketorolac for acute pain postsurgery Benefit has been shown when added to an opioid in WHO Step 3	Avoid in renal failure, GI bleeding, platelet abnormality, concomitant angiotensin converting enzyme inhibitory therapy, congestive heart failure; risk of drug interactions with anticoagulants and corticosteroids
Ibuprofen (PO)	25 min	1.8–2.5 h	400 mg q4 h (max 2.4 gm/day)	More effective for cancer pain associated with inflammation	
Ketamine	30–40 sec	2–3 h	Loading dose: 0.1–0.5 mg/kg Maintenance dose: 0.05–0.4 mg/kg/h	May decrease doses of concurrently used opioids; provides analgesia and sedation as a "dissociative anesthetic"; the treatment of chronic cancer pain not controlled by opioids or opioids plus adjuvant analgesics	Mild to severe emergence reactions (e.g., confusion, excitement, irrational behavior, hallucinations, delirium) [rare]; hypertension; arrhythmias
Steroids	N/A	N/A	Dexamethasone 2–8 mg oral, IV, or	Useful at any step in the WHO analgesic	Gastrointestinal bleeding; increase risk of infection;

Drug/Class	Onset of action	$t_{½}$	Dosing	Place in therapy	Common toxicities/major precautions
*Dexamethasone most often prescribed because it causes less fluid retention due to its lower mineralocorticoid effect			SQ q8 h Prednisone 7.5–10 mg daily	ladder when pain is due to edema or inflammation such as metastatic bone pain, neuropathic, and visceral pain	increased blood pressure; metabolic abnormalities; psychiatric disturbances; increased appetite, weight gain; insomnia Regimens should be tapered rather than abruptly discontinued if therapy exceeds 2 weeks
Gabapentin (PO)	N/A	5–7 h	Starting dose=100 mgTID 900–3600 mg/day in three divided doses	Neuropathic pain	CNS depression (common); confusion; ataxia; adjust dose in renal impairment; abrupt discontinuation associated with drug withdrawal syndrome; seizures; adjust for renal impairment
Carbamazepine (PO)	4–5 h	26–65 h, then 12–17 h	Starting dose = 50–100 mg BID; 100–200 mg q4–6 h (max 1200 mg/day)	Neuropathic pain	Somnolence (common); nystagmus; lethargy; Stevens-Johnson syndrome (rare); toxic epidermal necrolysis; agranulocytosis; adjust for CrCl <10 or hemodialysis; caution with hepatic impairment

PO, by mouth; IM, intramuscular; IV, intravenous; CrCl, creatinine clearance; BID, twice daily; TID, three times daily; APAP, acetaminophen; $t_{½}$, half-life of elimination; SQ, subcutaneous; CRRT, continuous renal replacement therapy; q, every; N/A, non-applicable; GI, gastrointestinal; CNS, central nervous system.

Table 5. Comparison of major non-opioid analgesic classes [4,20–23].

2.4. Unconventional modes of administration

Breathlessness is often a distressing symptom in oncology patients especially during end of life. Alternative routes of opioid administration, via inhaled nebulization and intranasal, have been studied. Unfortunately, data are still lacking on the efficacy of such routes of administration. However, benefit has been seen due to the short onset of action with these modes of delivery. Both morphine and fentanyl have been administered through nebulization, and fentanyl is preferred intranasally due its lipophilic properties allowing for better absorption [21].

2.5. Protocolized management of pain

In mechanically ventilated patients, use of protocols can greatly reduce the delay in treating pain, ICU length of stay, high dose analgesics, and duration of mechanical ventilation. It is advised to initiate orders that allow nurses to select the appropriate dose of an analgesic agent based on the pain scale score. Minimal data exist on the incremental doses that should be administered with various pain scores. However, orders for the analgesic agent of choice have been applied to our current practice in an oncology ICU and proven to be effective which are listed as follows:

- Fentanyl 25 mcg IV every 15 min as needed for numeric pain score 1–2, critical pain observation tool (CPOT) 0–2, and/or Richmond agitation-sedation scale (RASS) +1.
- Fentanyl 50 mcg IV every 15 min as needed for numeric pain score 3–4, CPOT 3–4, and/or RASS +2.
- Fentanyl 75 mcg IV every 15 min as needed for numeric pain score 5–7, CPOT 5–6, and/or RASS +3.
- Fentanyl 100 mcg IV every 15 min as needed for numeric pain score 8–10, CPOT 7–8, and/or RASS +4.

Initial doses are defaulted but can be changed by the prescriber if more aggressive or more conservative doses are needed.

Pain should be assessed routinely especially after analgesic agents are administered. Most nursing standards expect pain to be reassessed within 15–30 min after treatment, and thus, the frequency of analgesic medications should be written to allow redosing in a timely manner if needed [4].

3. Analgesia-First Sedation

Recent literature now emphasizes the importance of adequately treating pain prior to use of sedatives. The most common source of agitation identified in intubated patients is pain. If agitation is treated immediately with sedatives, then the patient is at risk of experiencing the physiologic consequences previously discussed because pain remains untreated. Therefore, it may be beneficial to have intermittent analgesic medication orders written to PRN RASS scores in addition to incremental pain scores to allow the nurse to adequately use such medications for agitation (as shown in example above).

If pain is ruled out as the cause of agitation, then other causes should be promptly considered such as hypoxemia, hypoglycemia, hypotension, or withdrawal from alcohol or other drugs [4]. Aside from treating such underlying causes, strategies should be used to help reduce agitation by maintaining comfort for the patient, frequent reorientation, and optimization of the environment to maintain normal sleep patterns. After addressing such issues, sedatives only then should be considered if the patient remains agitated with a goal sedation level established: light for goals of extubation (i.e. the patient is alert, calm, arousable, and able to follow commands) or deep sedation with goals of synchronization with the ventilator, or the prevention of movement in severe trauma/burns/paralysis (i.e. patient is unresponsive to painful stimuli, unable to follow commands) with goals of synchronization with the ventilator, or the prevention of movement severe trauma/burns). Most patients should have goals of light sedation as many studies have demonstrated increased ICU length of stay, mechanical ventilation, delirium, and muscle deconditioning with deep, prolonged sedation [25–27].

Agitation should be assessed as frequently as pain is assessed using the RASS or SAS scales (**Tables 6** and **7**). Recommendations for options to treat agitation are in **Table 8**.

Scale	Label	Description
+4	Combative	Combative, violent
+3	Very agitated	Pulls to remove tubes or catheters; aggressive
+2	Agitated	Frequent nonpurposeful movement, fights ventilator
+1	Restless	Anxious, apprehensive, movements not aggressive
0	Alert and calm	Spontaneously pays attention to caregiver
−1	Drowsy	Not fully alert, but has sustained awakening to voice (eye opening & contact >10 s)
−2	Light sedation	Briefly awakens to voice (eyes open & contact < 10 s)
−3	Moderate sedation	Movement or eye opening to voice (no eye contact)
−4	Deep sedation	No response to voice, but movement or eye opening to physical stimulation
−5	Unarousable	No response to voice or physical stimulation

Table 6. Richmond agitation sedation scale (RASS) [28].

Score	Term	Descriptor
7	Dangerous agitation	Pulling at ET tube, trying to remove catheters, climbing over bedrail, striking at staff, thrashing side to side
6	Very agitated	Requiring restraint and frequent verbal reminding of limits, biting ET tube
5	Agitated	Anxious or physically agitated, calms to verbal instructions
4	Calm and cooperative	Calm, easily arousable, follows commands
3	Sedated	Difficult to arouse but awakens to verbal stimuli or gentle shaking, follow simple commands but drifts off again

Score	Term	Descriptor
2	Very sedated	Arouses to physical stimuli but does not communicate or follow commands, may move spontaneously
1	Unarousable	Minimal or no response to noxious stimuli, does not communicate or follow commands ET, endotracheal.

Table 7. Sedation agitation scale [29].

Drug/MOA	Onset of action	$t_{½}$	Effects	Dosing	Place in therapy	Common toxicities/major precautions
Dexmedetomidine Selective α_2-agonist	5–10 min	1.8–3.1 h	Anxiolytic, sedative, analgesic/opioid sparing	Bolus: 1 mcg/kg over 10 min. Infusion: 0.2–0.7 mcg/kg/h	Assists in keeping patient calm and arousable to wean off the ventilator or for the treatment of acute hyperactive delirium; causes minimal respiratory depression	**Common:** bradycardia and hypotension, hypertension with loading dose. **Rare:** loss of airway reflexes, risk for withdrawal after prolonged (7 days) use. Infusion must be tapered slowly to prevent rebound agitation; slower emergence with hepatic failure
Propofol Binds to $GABA_A$, glycine, nicotinic, and M_1 muscarinic receptors	1–2 min	26–32 h	Sedative, hypnotic, anxiolytic, amnestic, antiemetic, anticonvulsant	Bolus: 5 mcg/kg/min Infusion: 5–50 mcg/kg/min	Light or heavy sedation; ideal for neurosurgery patients to allow for daily neurological assessments or medical ICU patients requiring deep sedation for vent synchronization; treatment of seizures and elevated intracranial pressure	Hypotension; respiratory depression; hypertriglyceridemia (with prolonged use), rhabdomyolysis (rare), pancreatitis (rare), deep sedation with propofol is associated with longer emergence times; lipid emulsion delivering 1.1 kcal/mL
Midazolam Activate γ-aminobutyric acid A ($GABA_A$) neuronal receptors	2–5 min	3–11 h	Sedative, hypnotic, anxiolytic, amnestic, antiemetic, anticonvulsant	1–14 mg/h (max ~0.1 mg/kg/h)	Patients requiring deep sedation; treatment of seizures or alcohol withdrawal	Respiratory depression; hypotension; accumulates in hepatic dysfunction; active metabolite accumulates in renal dysfunction; drug has potential to accumulate in adipose

http://dx.doi.org/10.5772/64268

Drug/MOA	Onset of action	$t_{½}$	Effects	Dosing	Place in therapy	Common toxicities/major precautions
						tissue with continuous infusions
Lorazepam Activate γ-aminobutyric acid A (GABA A) neuronal receptors	15–20 min	8-15 h	Sedative, hypnotic, anxiolytic, amnestic, antiemetic, anticonvulsant	1–10 mg/h	Patients requiring deep sedation; treatment of seizures or alcohol withdrawal	Respiratory depression; hypotension; propylene glycol-related acidosis (rare); nephrotoxicity evident by an osmolar gap greater than 10–12 mOsm/L; accumulates in hepatic dysfunction; emergence from lorazepam after prolonged infusions will be longer than midazolam due to its greater potency and slower clearance; drug has potential to accumulate in adipose tissue with continuous infusions

$t_{½}$, half-life of elimination; MOA, mechanism of action.

Table 8. Sedative agents [4,23,30].

4. Delirium

Delirium is defined as a syndrome with acute onset of cerebral dysfunction due to a change or fluctuation in baseline mental status, inattention, or disorganized thinking [4]. Two forms of delirium can exist: hyperactive (agitated, associated with hallucinations or delusions) or hypoactive (calm, lethargic, confused, and sedated). With delirium now being shown to be a strong predictor of negative long-term outcomes, it is imperative that regular assessments are performed to identify incidences of delirium and implementing preventative measures [24,31]. Such strategies include early mobilization, maintenance of light sedation while avoiding benzodiazepines in those with underlying risk factors for delirium, promoting sleep in adult ICU patients by optimizing environmental factors such as light, noise, clustering patient care activities, and decreasing stimuli at night.

Medication-induced delirium is not well studied and the exact onset, duration, or severity has yet to be confirmed. Delirium is multifactorial and, therefore, medications should not be solely considered as the cause in a patient experiencing changes in mental status. Most common causes of delirium are in **Table 9**. Benzodiazepines have been studied extensively as a possible risk factor for delirium. The data concerning benzodiazepines and outcomes with causing delirium remain controversial. The MENDS and SEDCOM studies had similar results showing higher delirium free days with or without coma when dexmedetomidine was administered compared to midazolam or lorazepam. Furthermore, both have similar results in showing no difference in mortality and the length of ICU stay [33,34]. However, another meta-analysis including six trials comparing benzodiazepine versus nonbenzodiazepine sedatives found opposite results. The ICU length of stay and duration of mechanical ventilation were significantly higher in the benzodiazepine group with no difference found in delirium prevalence or all-cause mortality [35]. Until further research can clarify such effects, caution is still warranted when using these sedatives and other risk factors shown in **Table 10** should be considered as well.

Iatrogenic	Exposure to sedative and opioid medications
Environmental	Prolonged physical restraints
	Immobilization
	Disorientation to time and space
Other	Drug or alcohol withdrawal
	Sepsis
Medication induced	Anticholinergics
	Benzodiazepines
	Opiates
	Antipsychotics
	Antispasmodics
	Anticonvulsants
	Corticosteroids

Table 9. Common causes of delirium [4,32].

Age
Pre-existing delirium
History of baseline hypertension
Sedative-associated coma
Mechanical ventilation
Polytrauma
Emergency surgery prior to ICU admission
APACHE II score
Metabolic acidosis
Delirium on the previous day

Table 10. Risk factors for delirium [36].

Two scales for assessing delirium with the highest psychometric (e.g., validity and reliability) scores are the CAM-ICU and the ICDSC [37]. Delirium should be assessed every 8–12 hours, only after sedatives are decreased or interrupted and preferably during daytime hours.

Drug	Usual starting dose/ available formulations	Short-term adverse effects		Additional considerations
		Low risk	Moderate to high risk	
Olanzapine	5 mg (PO, disintegrating tablet, IM)	EPS, NMS	Anticholinergic, weight gain, dyslipidemia	Increased risk of accumulation in elderly, female, and hepatic/ renal impairment; QT prolongation
Quetiapine	12.5–25 mg (PO)	NMS, weight gain, tardive dyskinesia, seizures, EPS	Anticholinergic (dry mouth, constipation), sedation, dizziness, Hypotension (with rapid titration), weight gain, dyslipidemia	Associated with lowest risk of EPS and tardive dyskinesia
Risperidone	0.5–1 mg (PO, disintegrating tablet)	Anticholinergic, NMS, cardiac conduction abnormalities	Orthostatic hypotension (with rapid titration),	EPS associated with doses >6 mg/day
Ziprasidone	20 mg PO 10 mg IM	Anticholinergic, sedation, EPS, NMS	QTc prolongation	IM formulation contains a nephrotoxin called cyclodextrin that can accumulate in renal impairment; reduce dose in hepatic impairment

PO, by mouth; IM, intramuscular; EPS, extrapyramidal symptoms; NMS, neuroleptic malignant syndrome.

Table 11. Atypical antipsychotics for the treatment of delirium [24,30,38,39].

Treatment of delirium should be directed at the probable underlying causes (e.g., alcohol or drug withdrawal, infection, dehydration, discomfort) and consider pharmacologic agents only if needed. SCCM guidelines provide a Grade C recommendation that "atypical antipsychotics may reduce the duration of delirium in adult ICU patients." No evidence exists on the efficacy of haloperidol in reducing delirium and is associated with higher incidences of extrapyramidal and cardiac side effects [38]. The atypical antipsychotics, which have been studied and shown to be beneficial, are listed in **Table 11**. If such agents are initiated, it is crucial to ensure they are discontinued upon discharge or follow-up strategies are in place in the outpatient setting. Patients should also be monitored carefully for the adverse effects listed.

The fundamental component of implementing successful protocols to manage pain, agitation, and delirium in mechanically ventilated patients is a multidisciplinary team. Developing a comprehensive protocol can help reduce costs, improve ICU outcomes, and create more consistent practices. As presented earlier, the SCCM PAD Guideline concepts can be employed but the basic principles established in cancer patients for managing pain and anxiety must also be considered to achieve optimal outcomes.

Author details

Trisha Patel* and Mark E. Lewis

*Address all correspondence to: trisha.patel@ctca-hope.com

Cancer Treatment Centers of America at Eastern Regional Medical Center, Philadelphia, USA

References

[1] Soares M, Depuydt PO. Mechanical ventilation in cancer patients: clinical characteristics and outcomes. Crit Care Clin. 2010; 26:41–58.

[2] Nelson JE, Meier DE, et al. Self-reported symptom experience of critically-ill cancer patients receiving intensive care. Crit Care Med. 2001; 29:277–282.

[3] Ripamonti CI, Bandieri E, et al. Management of cancer pain: ESMO Clinical Practice Guidelines. Ann Oncol. 2011; 22 (Suppl. 6):vi69–vi77.

[4] Barr J, Fraser GL, Puntillo K, et al. Clinical practice guidelines for the management of pain, agitation, and delirium in adult patients in the intensive care unit. Crit Care Med. 2013; 41:263–306.

[5] Stites M. Observational pain scales in critically ill adults. Crit Care Nurse. 2013; 33(3): 68–79.

[6] Beutler AS. Cancer pain. Retrieved January 01, 2016, from http://www.mayo.edu/research/labs/chronic-pain/cancer-pain.

[7] Dumas EO, Pollack GM. Opioid tolerance development: a pharmacokinetic/pharmacodynamic perspective. AAPS J. 2008; 10(4):537–551.

[8] Yu X. Analgesic management of chronic pain patients in the ICU. ICU Dir Clin Rev. 2013; 4(5):217–222.

[9] Mary Lynn M. *Update to Demystifying Opioid Conversion Calculations: A Guide for Effective Dosing*. Bethesda, MD: American Society of Health-System Pharmacists, 2009.Web.

[10] McPherson ML. Demystifying Opioid Conversion Calculations: A Guide for Effective Dosing. Bethesda, MD, USA: ASHP, 2009. ProQuest ebrary. Web. 3 February 2016.

[11] NCCN Clinical Practice Guidelines: Adult Cancer Pain. Version 2.2016. Retrieved from: https://www.nccn.org/professionals/physician_gls/pdf/pain.pdf

[12] Puntillo KA, White C, et al. Patients' perceptions and responses to procedural pain: results from Thunder Project II. Am J Crit Care. 2001; 10(4):238–251.

http://dx.doi.org/10.5772/64268

[13] Erstad BL, Puntillo K, et al. Pain management principles in the critically ill. CHEST. 2009; 135:1075–1086.

[14] Jacobi J, Fraser GL, et al. Clinical practice guidelines for the sustained use of sedatives and analgesics in the critically ill adult. Crit Care Med. 2002; 30 (1):119–141.

[15] Ketorolac Tromethamine injection [package insert]. Schaumburg, IL: Sagent Pharmaceuticals; revised 2/2014.

[16] Orirmev ® (acetaminophen) [package insert]. Hazelwood, MO: Mallinckrodt Pharmaceuticals; revised 12/2014.

[17] Argoff CE, Silvershein DI. A comparison of long- and short-acting opioids for the treatment of chronic noncancer pain: tailoring therapy to meet patient needs. Mayo Clin Proc. 2009; 84(7):602–612.

[18] DOLOPHINE® HYDROCHLORIDE CII (Methadone Hydrochloride Tablets, USP) [package insert]. Columbus, OH: Roxane Laboratories, Inc. Revised October 2006.

[19] Dworkin RH, O'Connor AB, et al. Pharmacologic management of neuropathic pain: evidence-based recommendations. Pain. 2007; 132:237–251.

[20] Acetaminophen (paracetamol): Drug Information. In:UpToDate. Lexicomp. Accessed on December 10, 2015.

[21] Bausewein C, Simon ST. Inhaled nebulized and intranasal opioids for the relief of breathlessness. Curr Opin Support Palliat Care. 2014; 8:208–212.

[22] Vyvey M. Steroids as pain relief adjuvants. Palliative Care Files. Can Fam Phys. 2010; 56:1295–1297.

[23] Riker RR, Fraser GL. Adverse effects associated with sedatives, analgesics, and other drugs that provide patient comfort in the intensive care unit. Pharmacotherapy. 2005; 25(5 Pt 2):8S–18S.

[24] Czosnowski QA, Whitman CB. Sedatives, analgesics, and neuromuscular blockage in the ICU. In: Roberts PR, Todd SR, editors. Comprehensive Critical Care: Adult. Mount Prospect: Society of Critical Care Medicine; 2012. pp. 759–778.

[25] Tanaka LS, Azevedo LP, et al. Early sedation and clinical outcomes of mechanically ventilated patients: a prospective multicenter cohort study. Crit Care. 2014; 18(R156): 1–10.

[26] Treggiari MM, Romand JA, et al. Randomized trial of light versus deep sedation on mental health after critical illness. Crit Care Med. 2009; 37:2527–2534.

[27] Kollef MH, Levy NT, et al. The use of continuous IV sedation is associated with prolongation of mechanical ventilation. CHEST 1998; 114:541–548.

[28] Sessler CN, Gosnell MS, et al. The Richmond agitation–sedation scale. Am J Respir Crit Care Med. 2002; 166(10):1338–1344.

[29] Riker RR, Picard JT, Fraser GL. Prospective evaluation of the sedation-agitation scale for adult critically ill patients. Crit Care Med. 1999; 27:1325–1329.

[30] Tietze K, Fuchs B. Sedative-analgesic medications in critically ill adults: Properties, dosage regimens, and adverse effects. In: UpToDate, Parsons PE (Ed), Waltham, MA: UpToDate. Accessed on February 25, 2016.

[31] Boogaard M, Schoonhoven L. et al. Delirium in critically ill patients: impact on long-term health-related quality of life and cognitive functioning. Crit Care Med. 2012; 40:112–118.

[32] Schreiber MP, Colantuoni E. et al. Corticosteroids and transition to delirium in patients with acute lung injury. Crit Care Med. 2014; 42:1480–1486.

[33] Riker RR, Shehabi Y, et al. Dexmedetomidine vs Midazolam for sedation of critically ill patients a randomized trial. JAMA. 2009; 301(5):489–499.

[34] Pandharipande PP, Pun BT, et al. Effect of sedation with dexmedetomidine vs lorazepam on acute brain dysfunction in mechanically ventilated patients. The MENDS randomized controlled trial. JAMA. 2007; 298 (22):2644–2653.

[35] Fraser GL, Devlin JW, et al. Benzodiazepine versus nonbenzodiazepine-based sedation for mechanically ventilated, critically ill adults: a systematic review and meta-analysis of randomized trials. Crit Care Med. 2013; 41:S30–S38.

[36] Zaal IJ, Devlin JW, et al. A systematic review of risk factors for delirium in the ICU. Crit Care Med. 2015; 43:40–47.

[37] Brummel NE, Vasilevskis EE. Implementing delirium screening in the ICU: secrets to success. Crit Care Med. 2013; 41:1–13.

[38] Haddad PM, Sharma SG. Adverse effects of atypical antipyschotics. Differential risk and clinical implications. CNS Drugs. 2007; 21(911):911–936.

[39] SEROQUEL (quetiapine) [package insert]. Wilmington, DE: AstraZeneca Pharmaceuticals LP; 1997.